Methods for
cohort studies of
chronic airflow limitation

World Health Organization
Regional Office for Europe
Copenhagen

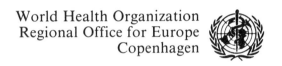

Methods for cohort studies of chronic airflow limitation

C. du V. Florey

Department of Community Medicine
St Thomas's Hospital Medical School
London, United Kingdom

and

S.R. Leeder

Faculty of Medicine
University of Newcastle
New South Wales, Australia

WHO Regional Publications, European Series No. 12

This publication is dedicated to the memory of David Maddison, late Dean of the Faculty of Medicine at the University of Newcastle, NSW, who provided inspiration to the many members of the Faculty, and especially to the authors during the preparation of the book.

ISBN 92 890 1103 3

TYPESET IN INDIA
PRINTED IN ENGLAND

CONTENTS

ACKNOWLEDGEMENTS

We should like to take this opportunity of thanking the many people who gave advice. In particular, we thank Associate Professor A. J. Woolcock for her comments and for providing Annex 6 describing the test for bronchial reactivity. We also thank Miss S. Chinn, Dr A. Dobson, Professor W. W. Holland, Dr M. Karvonen, Professor P. Macklem, Mr A. Swan and Dr R. van der Lende for their searching and most constructive criticism. Mr Swan also kindly provided Fig. 2. We are very grateful to Mrs Terese Alder for the many patient hours spent typing and retyping the manuscript.

C. du V. Florey is also grateful to the Faculty of Medicine, University of Newcastle, New South Wales, Australia, for providing support during his sabbatical leave, when this book was written.

Introduction

With the advent of antibiotics in the 1940s the importance of acute respiratory infections as a cause of morbidity and high mortality declined rapidly. However in some countries, particularly the United Kingdom, the burden of chronic disease of the respiratory system has persisted, with substantial death rates ascribed to "chronic bronchitis". Because of the importance of chronic respiratory conditions as a cause of lost productivity, lower quality of life, and a drain on health service resources, a large number of studies have been carried out to investigate their etiology in a search for methods of prevention and a more precise definition of their natural history.

The search for a working definition of chronic lung disease started with the term "chronic non-specific lung disease" (1). This was then superseded by "chronic obstructive lung disease" and "chronic airways obstruction". Recently it has been suggested (2) that the term "chronic airflow limitation" best describes the common problem of patients with a number of underlying abnormalities, including emphysema, bronchiolitis, chronic bronchitis and chronic asthma. Emphysema is enlargement of the distal air spaces accompanied by the destruction of alveolar walls, and bronchiolitis is inflammation, obstruction or obliteration of the bronchioles. Both conditions can be diagnosed with certainty only on biopsy or at autopsy. Chronic bronchitis, better described as mucus hypersecretion, is characterized by chronic sputum production, and the term should be used specifically for this clinical situation; by itself it does not necessarily cause airflow limitation. Patients with long-standing, severe asthma may have chronic airflow limitation due to residual obstruction, the pathology of which is poorly understood but includes smooth muscle hypertrophy and bronchiolitis with mucus plugging.

Chronic airflow limitation may be partially reversible in response to bronchodilator treatment in some patients, but the term implies that, in spite of maximal therapy, there is residual limitation to airflow on forced expiration. There is no agreement as to which test best demonstrates the inability to blow air rapidly from the lungs. However, it is generally recognized that the volume/flow/time relations of a

1

forced expiration will reveal established abnormalities causing airflow limitation and possibly also subtle changes when the underlying abnormalities are at an early stage.

Etiological factors found to be related to chronic airflow limitation include, most importantly, cigarette smoking and high levels of particulate air pollution from industrial, domestic and occupational sources. Chronic airflow limitation also occurs more frequently in males than in females at all ages. It is a major health problem, especially in older people, when the clinical manifestations become serious, demanding increasing medical care and causing absenteeism from work.

Despite the large number of studies of chronic airflow limitation, many questions remain unanswered. We do not know what the origins of the obstruction are. Does the process start in childhood? Indirect evidence suggests that it does, but detailed long-term studies have not yet been carried out. Does it spring from susceptibility to viral infection in the first two years of life, or is there another, endogenous, factor that is switched on by viral infection? Can the potential patient be identified in time to prevent disease?

From another point of view, the effects of environmental pollution may be monitored or examined through changes in, or contrasts between, respiratory illness rates of people exposed to different concentrations of the pollutants concerned. This approach may be used to study either acute episodes of pollution suspected of having long-term effects, or chronic lower levels of pollution. Opportunities for such studies arise wherever there is industrial development. Epidemiological studies are essential whenever there is a catastrophe in which chemicals are released that may have long-term consequences for the health of the exposed population.

But why is an epidemiological approach needed? Studies on animals have contributed substantially to the understanding of the effects of a variety of factors on the respiratory system. However, the results are not directly applicable to man because of species differences and because, in most studies, the concentrations required to elicit a response within a reasonably short space of time have been far in excess of those experienced by human populations in the general environment. Laboratory experiments on human volunteers, in which control over the levels of factors of specific interest allows precise estimates of exposure to be made, have also contributed, but have been limited because of ethical and practical considerations; in particular, they are rarely conducted under natural conditions.

Since definitive answers to many of the problems posed by chronic airflow limitation have not been forthcoming from animal or human laboratory experiments, epidemiological studies have played a major part in defining the roles of putative causes.

This publication describes the epidemiological methods for studying the evolution of chronic airflow limitation, and is a contribution to the WHO programme for the control of chronic diseases. The investigation of the origins of respiratory illness has been strongly supported by

WHO in the past through its sponsorship of a multinational study of the relation between air pollution and respiratory symptoms and disease in primary school children, but there is now a need to develop a general methodology for research on chronic airflow limitation. This need has also been recognized by the WHO European regional programme on environmental health aspects of the control of chemicals, in which a multifaceted approach to environmental problems has been used. As one part of that programme, epidemiological investigations are to be carried out to study the toxicity of groups of chemicals in specific situations or from specific sources.

More experience has probably been gained worldwide in the epidemiological investigation of chronic airflow limitation through studies of the effects of air pollution, including tobacco smoke, than of any other risk factor. A variety of study designs and measurements of the respiratory system have been used, so that it is now possible to describe a general plan and the options within it for studies of factors predictive of chronic airflow limitation. Furthermore, considerable experience has already been gained of international cooperative studies in the field, so that their strengths and weaknesses are well known (even if the solutions to some of the problems are not yet clear). It is our purpose to identify the successful methods from past work and to describe how a cohort study of the evolution of chronic lung disease might be conducted.

The aim of this book is to assist research workers in the design and execution of their own studies of chronic airflow limitation. Chapter 1 is concerned with the general design of cohort studies, and with their advantages and disadvantages in comparison with other epidemiological methods. The foundations are laid here, but further introductory reading will be essential for readers unfamiliar with the epidemiological approach. In Chapter 2 we discuss the types of population suitable for study and the difficulties of interpreting the data obtained from them. Chapter 3 covers in detail the methods of obtaining a history of respiratory illness and of measuring lung function. It emphasises the need for simplicity and for the rejection of complex measurements, which are unreliable in the field. Chapter 4 describes the statistical analysis of the data. This is not comprehensive—the mark of the good research worker is the ability to marshal the data in unusual patterns to give insight into a problem—but it sets out the essential basic approaches and draws attention to the analytical power provided by the relatively new computer programs for generalized linear models. Chapter 5 deals with documentation, and stresses the importance of the protocol.

All the methods described have been tested in the field and are known to work in principle. They will need modification and adaptation to local situations. Their ultimate success in helping to unravel the remaining questions posed by chronic airflow limitation will depend on the skill of the investigator.

CHAPTER 1

Principles of epidemiological studies

Most epidemiological studies make use of naturally occurring situations rather than designed experiments, and several methods have been developed to take advantage of such situations. The simplest approach to the investigation of problems in the community is *descriptive*: the characteristics of people and of their environment are counted or measured and their frequency or some statistical quantity is used to portray the situation. This is a sound approach in the early stages of an epidemic of an infectious disease or when the health of a community is being mapped in order to assist in planning the delivery of services. Plotting the variations in mortality by month or year of birth is another example. The data may also be used to suggest hypotheses.

ANALYTICAL STUDIES

A somewhat more complex approach is that of analytical studies, in which hypotheses may be generated from the results of a variety of analyses of the interrelations between variables, or hypotheses may be tested in suitable naturally occurring circumstances or in the contrived circumstances of an experiment. Four general designs are used in epidemiological studies: the cross-sectional, the case-control, the randomized controlled and the cohort. The last is our concern here, but a brief review of the first two will show how they relate in practical terms to the cohort study. (The randomized controlled trial is a highly specialized design and is not considered here.)

Cross-sectional studies

The cross-sectional study is one in which selected attributes of a population (or a sample of the population) are measured at one point in time. The data may be used purely descriptively, to show how much of some measured characteristic there is in the population, or to help to develop hypotheses. The frequency of qualitative characteristics (such as symptoms or diseases) is usually given as a prevalence rate (the number of people with the characteristic divided by the number of people examined or, alternatively, in the sample). Quantitative characteristics, such as vital capacity, can be expressed in the form of histograms or in terms of their means and standard deviations. Cross-sectional studies may also be analytical, since the interrelations between the variables can be examined. Hypotheses of cause and effect and of association can be developed from an assessment of the relations between variables. However, the design allows only the *testing* of rather simple hypotheses, e.g. does the prevalence rate or the mean of some characteristic differ from some selected value or from the values obtained in other populations? Even these "tests" lead only to further hypotheses to explain any difference found. This limitation of the design – namely, that the studies do not provide the data for determining the direction of influence between correlated variables – stems from the fact that the sample is composed of survivors of some original but unspecified cohort, the remainder having emigrated or died, and from the lack of data from the past to determine the order of events in a cause-and-effect model. For data obtained by recall, this problem may be partially overcome, but the reliability of the information must be suspect.

Case-control studies

The case-control design is used for testing hypotheses of cause and effect. Both the cause and the effect must be specified in advance so that at least two groups, one with and the other without the effect (or disease), may be questioned to determine whether or to what extent the putative cause was encountered in the past. This is the design frequently used in clinical epidemiological studies, because both cases and controls can be drawn from hospital patients, and details of past events may be obtained either during a consultation for other purposes or from written records. The speed of execution and the need only for small numbers of observations, as compared with the cross-sectional or cohort studies (an obvious advantage for the study of rare diseases), make this design particularly attractive. However, there are many drawbacks because of biases that can affect the results.

These biases have been described by Sackett (*3*) and are mentioned briefly here because some of them are applicable to cohort studies (most can, however, be avoided in such studies provided that their existence is appreciated). The major biases can be divided into those that affect the sampling and those that affect the measurement, either of the event or condition, or of the predisposing factor.

Prevalence–incidence bias

This bias (*4*) is encountered in all epidemiological studies. It relates to the effect on the analysis of people missing from the sample because they failed to survive long enough to take part, their episodes of illness were too short to be recorded during the survey, evidence for their exposure to the causal factors was lost, or the condition, though present, was clinically silent. Some of these people never appear in the sample because of the consequences of the severity of their condition, thereby probably weakening the association with the causal factor, whereas others with the condition may be placed in the control group because of failure to diagnose. Failure to determine past exposure will affect the correct classification of cases and controls and may bias the result in an unmeasurable way, either in favour of or against an association.

Admission rate bias

This bias (5) relates to the effect of different entry rates into the sample of people in the four basic categories (case, control, exposed, non-exposed). This is simply illustrated by a theoretical example. It might be of interest to see whether chronic bronchitis (CB) and carcinoma of the lung (CaL) tend to be mutually exclusive conditions. In some defined population of 4000 people, let us suppose that 15 % have CB and 10 % have CaL and that the two diseases are independent. Of the 600 people with CB, 60 (10 %) have CaL and of the 3400 people without CB, 340 (also 10 %) have CaL. If the mortality rates (which may be thought of as admission rates to post-mortem examination) are 40 % for CB, 80 % for CaL and 20 % for "not CB", the pathologist will find that 53/269 people with CB have CaL (19.7 %) and 286/898 "not CB" people will have CaL (31.9 %). The chi-square value (14.2) indicates that the difference in the percentages is extremely unlikely to have occurred by chance ($P < 0.001$), which points to a protective effect of CB for CaL, whereas the truth is that the two diseases are independent of each other. Since there is no way of preventing this bias in case-control studies, nor can it be measured, the value of the results of a single study or of several using the same technique is limited. The calculations are illustrated in Tables 1–3.

Table 1. Distribution of chronic bronchitics (CB), lung cancer patients (CaL) and those without these conditions ($\overline{CB}$, $\overline{CaL}$) in a general population of 4000 people

	CB	$\overline{CB}$	Total
CaL	60	340	400
$\overline{CaL}$	540	3060	3600
Total	600	3400	4000
With CaL	10.0 %	10.0 %	

No association between CB and CaL.

Table 2. Calculation of deaths from CB plus CaL (given independence of effects).
Mortality rates: CB = 40%; CaL = 80%; $\overline{CB}$ = 20%

CaL	CB		
	Alive	Dead	Total
Alive	7	5	} 53
Dead	29	19	
Total	36	24	60

Of the 60 people with CB and CaL, 40% die of CB. Of the 36 remaining, 80% die of CaL. A similar calculation for the 340 people with CaL and $\overline{CB}$ yields 286 deaths.

Table 3. Numbers coming to post-mortem. Mortality rates: CB = 40%; CaL = 80%; $\overline{CB}$ = 20%

	CB	$\overline{CB}$	Total
CaL	53	286	339
$\overline{CaL}$	216	612	828
Total	269	898	1167
With CaL	19.7%	31.9%	

Highly significant negative association between CB and CaL.

Unmasking bias

This bias arises when the factor under consideration is innocent but causes a symptom of the disease in question that leads to the unmasking of the disease through subsequent clinical investigation. In other words, some of the cases may be detected because their contact with the factor caused them to have symptoms of their disease, not because the factor caused the disease. Since the cases and controls are selected by different processes (only one of which includes provocation by the factor) they cease to be suitable for comparison (6). Thus exposure to an occupational factor causing wheezing, but not asthma, may lead to investigations that "unmask" a group of latent asthmatics, who are then

8

classed together with other asthmatics discovered in the normal way. Exposure to the occupational factor may then be found more frequently among the cases than in the non-asthmatic control population. This bias tends to increase the perceived strength of association between the case condition and the "cause". It may be prevented by matching cases and controls on the method of detection, though this can lead to overmatching so that a real effect is missed.

Non-response bias

The effects of this bias on the results cannot readily be predicted, but characteristics of the non-responders can sometimes be obtained from other sources and compared with those of the responders to give clues as to its strength. Assessment of the bias may also be possible by selecting a random sample of the non-responders (to reduce the number of subjects involved) and seeking their cooperation with particular diligence.

Membership bias

This, the last of the major sampling biases, is caused by non-random allocation of cases and controls into groups exposed and not exposed to factors believed to be causative. The name is derived from the fact that the members of each group have themselves selected their exposure to factors such as cigarette smoking, physical exercise or dietary indiscretions. This bias cannot be prevented but evidence can be obtained to show whether there are important differences between the groups (such as age) that might lead to inappropriate conclusions.

Diagnostic suspicion bias

Measurement biases in case-control studies are mostly peculiar to that particular design, but the diagnostic suspicion bias may also occur in cohort studies. This bias arises when, in the course of investigation, either in an interview or in the assessment of physical or laboratory measurements, the investigator becomes suspicious of a respondent's diagnosis. This may lead him to order further investigations or be influenced in his interpretation in a non-standard way. Provided the existence of this bias is appreciated, the study can be designed to eliminate it by using "blind" techniques for assessment.

Calculation of relative risk

On the assumption that the biases have been avoided or accounted for in some way, the data from case-control studies may be used to calculate relative risk. This is the ratio of two absolute risks, the first being that of contracting the condition when exposed to the suspected causal factor and the second that of contracting the condition in the absence of the factor. Only the relative risk can be obtained from case-control studies and this only when the condition in the general population is rare (say $< 1\%$) and the cases and controls are representative of their respective populations (the derivation of relative risk or relative odds is treated in many elementary textbooks of statistics, such as that of Hills (7). Case-control studies do not provide the data necessary for the derivation of absolute risk, a statistic of greater interest since it indicates how frequently the condition occurs after exposure, without reference to any other group.

The disadvantages of case-control studies clearly make them unsuitable for drawing definitive conclusions about cause and effect. They are, however, valuable as a first step in testing hypotheses because of their practical simplicity and rapid execution. For very rare diseases they may be the only feasible, though not the ideal, design.

It might be well to remember the comment made on case-control studies by William Farr, first Superintendent of the Statistical Department in the General Register Office in England and Wales: "the replies will be general, vague and I fear of little value". It is essential to use cohort studies to test the results obtained from case-control studies whenever the problem is of sufficient importance to warrant the time and expense.

Cohort studies

A cohort is used here to mean a group of people defined at some point in time by certain characteristics, such as age, sex, race, or geographical location. For example, a cohort might be defined as all infants born in a country between specified dates (a birth cohort), or a group of 50-year-old executives living in Paris. If the cohort is randomly selected from the population with the defining characteristics, any observations made on it are referable to that population.

The aim of the cohort study is to determine whether characteristics observed at the start or appearing during the course of the study are related to subsequent events, such as myocardial infarction or death from respiratory illness. The study may start with a cohort of people who show no evidence of the disease or diseases of interest. This healthy cohort is obtained from a sample of unselected people by using the results of an examination to exclude those with disease. It is wise, however, to follow those who are excluded, because the results of their examinations may provide insight into the natural history of advanced disease that the healthy group cannot provide for many years. The data for the diseased group and the healthy cohort can be analysed separately without prejudice to either. The first examination is similar to a cross-sectional study, but arrangements have to be made so that the respondents can be followed up at some future time(s). At each examination every attempt must be made to obtain a 100% response. At the first examination not less than 90% of those in the sample should be seen because some of them will fail to come to follow-up examinations as a consequence of death, departure or disinclination. So important is the maintenance of a high response rate for the success of a cohort study that special and sometimes costly methods of keeping in contact with the cohort members are required. These include, for example, an annual letter with reply-paid card to check changes of address, and the building up of a feeling among respondents of belonging to something special and worth while. The extent to which contact need be made between examinations depends very much on the type of population under study, its stability, its geographical boundaries, and the importance it attaches to the research.

Three variations on the basic cohort design have been used to reduce the length of time required and to overcome the problem of increasing non-response with time.

If poor follow-up response is expected, the use of routinely collected data may be helpful. It may be possible to obtain data on mortality, hospital admissions or sickness absence for members of the cohort. The cohort might be defined *retrospectively* by using employment records in an industry, and information from regular medical check-ups and on retirement and mortality. Provided that the data are of good quality, it is then only necessary to examine the cohort once—a final follow-up so to speak. Although this can be a much faster and cheaper approach than the truly prospective one, it suffers from lack of standardization of past measurement and of data on some variables of interest, thus limiting its usefulness. This retrospective cohort design may be altered so that, in place of a single final survey, the defined cohort is examined several times over the following years. Thus the length of time required for the study is reduced, as before, but a more precise definition of the changes during the latter part of the period is obtained.

The second variation consists of using several cohorts of different ages and following them for a defined period, so that the age of each cohort reaches that of the initial age of the next older cohort. For example, two groups of children aged five and ten years at the start of a study might be followed for five years. In this way a picture of the development of disease can be built up relatively rapidly. However, the assumption that changes observed in a younger cohort were also experienced earlier by an older cohort must be assessed in some way, such as by taking into account changes with time in other factors that may have affected the disease process. Although this design has the advantage of speed in execution, it may lead to erroneous conclusions about the evolution of disease because of differences in lifetime experiences of the cohorts. For example, the 10-year-olds in the hypothetical study mentioned above might have suffered from a particularly severe epidemic of influenza before the birth of the five-year-olds.

The third variation may be used when the non-response over the period of study is expected to be high. If the duration of the study is to be, say, 15 years but non-response is expected to be substantial after five years, three cohorts might then be used, the first to be followed for five years, the second for the next five years and the third for the last five years. To avoid the biases introduced by different life experiences, each successive cohort should have the same age and sex structure as the preceding cohort would have had in its sixth year if there had been 100% response throughout. Moreover, the second and subsequent cohorts should consist of people who have remained in the area (or industry, etc.) for the entire period of the study. This design suffers from the lack of continuity of measurement on the same person, but may be useful in monitoring the effects of changing environmental pollutant levels over long periods, for which continuity may be less critical than in studies of natural history.

The *incidence rate* is the statistic unique to cohort studies, and is defined as:

$$\frac{\text{Number of new cases occurring in a given period}}{\text{Number of people at risk for that period}}$$

This may be multiplied by ten raised to a suitable power to give a value greater than one (more appealing to the eye than a probability value) and may be expressed in terms of fixed periods, e.g. per week, month or year. For example, there may be 50 new cases of lower respiratory infection in 3000 schoolchildren in a three-month period. The incidence rate is then 50 cases per 3000 children per three months. This can be presented in a more standard form as follows:

$$\frac{50}{3000} \times 1000 = 16.67 \text{ per 1000 per quarter year}$$

If the incidence rate did not vary with time it could be expressed per month by dividing by 3, or per year by multiplying by 4. This rate can also be calculated for different subgroups of the cohort, defined by their initial or subsequent values of selected variables, so as to determine the size of the risk associated with those values. Relative risks for pairs of subgroups can be calculated from the incidence rates.

Incidence rates may give a fairly precise estimate of incidence for easily recognized and reliably diagnosed diseases, but are less precise for most chronic non-infectious diseases. These degenerative diseases may run a long silent course before they become clinically overt, so that it is difficult to pinpoint the time when a healthy person becomes a new case. Because of its indeterminate nature, a new case must be defined for the purposes of the study, and in the same way as in other studies, if comparisons are to be made. Diagnostic criteria must be specified. These define the presence of the disease in terms that can be measured in an epidemiological study – some diagnostic tests are too complex to apply to large numbers of people – but they should also be clinically relevant, so that the results of the study can be used by clinicians as well as by community physicians.

The advantage of the cohort study as compared with cross-sectional and case-control studies, apart from the estimation of incidence, is that the natural history of a disease can be studied. Causes may be disentangled from associated factors and the rate of evolution or remission can be estimated. The risk of developing a disease can be estimated for a variety of initial characteristics, and several types of outcome can be observed (such as mortality, a specified decrease in lung function, or the onset of acute bronchial infection). Controls do not, as in case-control studies, have to be selected as a special group with all the inherent biases, but may be chosen from the cohort itself according to the problem being tackled. The measurements and diagnoses can be made under strict control and by means of standardized techniques.

There are, however, certain disadvantages that must be weighed carefully before a cohort study is undertaken. Because the investigator has to wait for the disease to develop in his cohort, and in most situations only a small proportion of the cohort will be affected, the study may take many years to complete and large initial populations are required. The size and duration of the study make it expensive. Promise of financial support for the project until it is complete is needed, otherwise early work will be wasted if the outcome measures cannot be made.

Biases may affect the results of the study. The problem of non-response has been emphasized, and other *sampling* biases common to case-control and cohort studies have been mentioned, though these are mostly avoidable or measurable in cohort studies. There are a variety of *measurement* biases, one of which has already been mentioned (diagnostic suspicion) but, of these, the instrument bias is of particular concern. Instruments should obviously be properly calibrated and maintained so that they give accurate and reliable readings. However, in longitudinal studies, drift in calibration techniques or reference standards can lead to misinterpretation of time trends and the natural history of disease. It is essential to take precautions from the start to prevent the effects of this important bias. Allied to this is observer bias, which will change over time if different observers (laboratory technicians, interviewers, field-workers, etc.) are used from one examination to the next.

A cohort study is a major commitment. It requires a dedication not called for by the other study designs. The results may take years to appear and study personnel may change during that period. There must be at least one person in a senior position who will direct the work for the duration of the project and, for those coming to the study after it has started, documentation of a high standard, describing the method used, and the progress made, must be available. Good computing facilities are needed with appropriate staffing, including an experienced biostatistician. Of the three designs described here, the cohort study has the greatest potential for catastrophe but, given the will and the necessary financial support, it can be extremely rewarding.

Multiple cross-sectional studies

The difficulties of carrying out cohort studies have led to the use of a less demanding design in which repeated cross-sectional studies are carried out on random samples from the same population. This avoids the administrative complexity and cost of following up the same people. The design is superficially attractive but in no way has the properties of a true cohort study.

This multiple cross-sectional method has two purposes, first to show whether there are changes in prevalence from one survey to another associated with changes in risk-factor levels in the appropriate direction, and second, a special case of the first, to determine the effects of community intervention programmes. In the latter, the design has a particular advantage as compared with the cohort study in that the two (or more) samples of the population invited for examination are not influenced in their responses by the experience of previous examinations (the so-called Hawthorne effect) (8).

Because the multiple cross-sectional study has no follow-up, most of the advantages of the cohort study are lost. It is neither possible to describe the natural history nor estimate the incidence of disease, since what happens to individuals over time is not recorded. It is not possible to examine the results of subgroups—high-risk groups, for example—to determine which factors preceded and predisposed to clinical disease. Cause can be inferred, based on *a priori* knowledge, only if changes in risk-factor levels and in disease prevalence occur in the expected direction. However, the inference is subject to the biases outlined earlier, so that no definitive conclusions can be reached.

If the multiple cross-sectional design is used, certain practical considerations must be taken into account. The population under study must be very stable and no immigration or emigration of groups dissimilar in composition must take place. If the population is stable, random samples from it would be expected to yield results with predictable variability from one examination to another. If the population changes between examinations, however, any change in prevalence or factor levels may be due to those changes rather than to a real change in the levels of the original population. As a corollary, the sampling methods, the methods of data collection, and the response rate must clearly be comparable at each examination. It would be quite inappropriate, for example, to use interviewer-administered question-naires for one examination and postal questionnaires for another, or to compare prevalence rates between two examinations where the response rates were, say, 80% and 60%. (See the discussion of non-response bias on p. 9.)

It is unlikely that a general population will be completely stable over a period of several years, so that evidence must be obtained whereby the probability can be assessed that the changes in values between examin-ations are real, or are due to compositional changes in the population. It may be possible, before the analysis is started, to describe the expected changes for sub-groups. If an intervention programme to prevent cigarette smoking had been carried out between examinations, for example, it might then be hypothesized that the greatest effects would be in the young and the least in those over 60 years, who tend to be less

14

concerned with avoiding risks to life. If the pattern of change with age fits the hypothesis, it supports an effect of the programme. It is not proof, however, since the expected pattern may have been observed because of causally unconnected changes in the population. (In other words, if the two samples are drawn from a population that has changed with time, differences may be due to changes in the composition of the population rather than to secular changes or to changes due to an intervention in the original population.) Further evidence that the changes are not the result of bias may be found by comparing the frequency or mean values of variables that should not alter between surveys, such as age, sex or race. Variables used in defining the sample should not be used in these comparisons unless they cover a wide range of values. For example, if the samples were composed of males only, comparison of the frequency of males in the samples would be pointless, but if the samples contained people in the age range 20–64 years, comparison of the age frequency distributions might then be useful.

The design may be improved by including a small cohort that is seen at every examination. This cohort should be a random sample of the original population and of sufficient size to determine whether changes observed between cross-sectional samples are supported by similar changes in the cohort.

Sample sizes for multiple cross-sectional studies will be larger than for cohort studies, because the greater power of tests of differences between paired observations in the same individual cannot be exploited.

Despite their superficial similarity, the cohort and multiple cross-sectional studies serve different purposes. The choice of design for a particular investigation will depend both on the hypothesis and on the statistics required to test it.

STATISTICAL ANALYSIS

Cohort studies present particular difficulties in analysis because statistical theory has not been developed to the same extent for repeated observations on the same individuals as for observations made only once. The analytical procedure may therefore be divided into the following two major steps: (a) an analysis of the initial cross-sectional data; and (b) an analysis that takes into account the changes over the period of the study.

The data to be collected will depend on the hypothesis being tested (if there is no clearly defined hypothesis the study should never have been started). It is likely, however, that certain variables will be measured because they have been found important in previous studies. Obviously, measures of the functioning of the respiratory system will be needed, e.g. tests of lung function itself, measurement of phlegm production, and the frequency of respiratory symptoms and of treatment for named respiratory conditions. It is expected that the system will be affected by one or more environmental or genetic factors, some of which should be referred to in the hypothesis. They may include a new environmental hazard released by industry, a suspect biological agent, or time, a key factor in describing the natural history of a disease. In addition, there are confounding variables that are known to be associated with respiratory disease and the putative causal factors, and which may differ among individuals. If their effects are not taken into account differences in lung function may be attributed to the putative causal factors, when in fact they are due to related differences in the confounding variables.

In the first, cross-sectional survey, single observations on each variable will be made on each individual. After the data have been checked and corrected for punching and other errors, frequency distributions should be obtained for *every* variable. This permits a visual check of the ranges of the observations and is a reference document for any simple enquiries about the data. Cross-tabulations of some of the variables are needed for a broad assessment of associations, such as of lung function or symptom frequency with age and sex. A simple correlation analysis of continuously distributed variables will reveal *linear* trends (it is possible that curvilinear trends will not be detected in this way) that can be inspected in bivariate scatter diagrams. These descriptive analyses should give a feeling for the data, a prerequisite for any interpretation of more complex analyses.

A relational model is inherent in any epidemiological investigation. In the cohort study it takes the general form:

Suspect causative factor → Outcome in terms of human health

More specifically, this might be written in a conventional form in which the order is reversed:

Lung function = Particulate pollution

which may be read as "The variability in lung function between individuals may be explained (in part) by differences in exposure to particulate pollution". The outcome or dependent variable is conventionally written on the left-hand side of the equation.

The model may be expanded to include other factors on the right-hand side (independent variables). Some of these may be other causative agents and others may be confounding factors. A full model may need many variables to explain the variability in lung function, although there are practical limitations, e.g. the number should be substantially less than the number of people in the sample. Analyses of this sort help to disentangle the contribution of each independent variable to the prediction of lung function, after allowing for the effects of all the other variables in the model. An epidemiologist and a statistician should work together on the interpretation so as to obtain a balance between the biological and statistical relevance of the results.

The analyses can be used to describe the data and the interrelations between the variables on completion of the first examination. As the data are cross-sectional at this stage the primary hypotheses cannot be tested, but insight into the way the variables are distributed and correlated may be used to confirm or question the appropriateness of the sample for the investigation, and may indicate what modifications in follow-up examinations may be required.

Longitudinal analyses must assess the *changes* in the values of key variables in terms of their absolute values and of other factors. When small groups are involved, the changes may be plotted for each individual, but for larger groups summary statistics are required. Thus, in a study with only one follow-up examination, the significance of the change in the mean values of a given variable can be estimated for subgroups of the population after allowing for the effect of *regression to the mean (9–11)*. With more than one follow-up examination it may be possible to estimate the average change with time by regression methods and to use the regression coefficient as a single observation to describe the changes between multiple observations in an ordered series. Methods used in a longitudinal study of chronic respiratory disease (*12*) are referred to in Chapter 4.

USE OF COMPUTERS

Because of the complexity of the organization, execution and analysis of longitudinal studies, a computer is an essential "laboratory instrument". It may be used to store information on the population to be surveyed and to draw a suitable sample. It can hold the names and addresses of the sample members for purposes of follow-up letters and labelling of specimens. It must be used to check the examination data to ensure that all values are reasonable and that no inconsistencies occur. It is the best instrument for the accurate sorting and merging of data from different sources. It is effective in producing accurate counts of observations and is essential if the model-fitting analyses described briefly above are to be done (they cannot reasonably be done by hand). Because computers obey a set of instructions that can be recorded, the reasons for any errors found later can be traced much more easily than those made by humans.

A computer is involved at almost every stage of a study. Its effective use will depend on the skills of the statisticians in designing a reliable and flexible system of handling the data, and on good programming. Because the correct use of the computer is critical to the success of a study, it must be described in detail in the protocol at the beginning of the study. In this way, the questionnaire and measurement forms can be designed to ease transfer of data to the computer and to take advantage of whatever package and systems programs are available.

CHAPTER 2

Populations and sample size for cohort studies of respiratory illness

This chapter is concerned with populations that can be used for cohort studies. It is emphasized that the choice of population is highly dependent on the hypothesis to be tested. The advantages and disadvantages of populations defined by age, occupation, risk and family relationship are described. The second half of the chapter is devoted to the estimation of sample size and, albeit briefly, the concepts underlying the calculations are described. Although cohort studies present peculiar problems in sample size estimation that must be dealt with by a trained statistician, the underlying concepts are similar to those for simpler designs and should be mastered by the epidemiologist.

POPULATIONS

The population to be used in an epidemiological study is usually self-evident or easy to choose. It must, however, be appropriate to the hypothesis the study is designed to test. A wide variety of natural groupings of people exists, and it may be helpful to consider them and the kind of information that can be obtained about them.

In cohort studies of respiratory disease one may be investigating the evolution of the condition either under natural circumstances or after some preventive or therapeutic intervention. Here, the first step is to choose a suitable population from the many possible. The choice of population may be much more restricted, however, in an investigation of the respiratory consequences of exposure to an atmospheric pollutant occurring only in a small area. The population for study would then be defined by the boundaries within which the pollution occurs. An unexposed control population may be needed and its characteristics should match those of the exposed population.

A population for study may be defined by age, the youngest group consisting of newborn infants. Infants may be studied to identify potential risk factors developing in early life and predisposing to later chronic respiratory disease, and may easily be defined from a birth register, from which their usual place of residence should be available. There are unlikely to be any routinely collected statistics on the respiratory health of the children, although in some countries useful data may be obtained from clinic or general practitioner records. Common routine infant data recording systems, such as for immunization or congenital malformations, are not likely to be helpful in the study of respiratory illness. In this group, information on health should be collected specifically from the parents and medical attendants, and by physical examination by study personnel using standardized techniques (13).

Preschool children are similar to infants in that they constitute an appropriate group for use in a search for risk factors for respiratory disease, but are particularly difficult to sample as, in many countries, there is no register of their names, addresses and ages. Those who go to crèche, playschool or kindergarten do not usually account for all children in this age range, so that sampling from these groups will not yield a group representative of all preschool children in an area. The small amount of work done on this age group reflects the difficulties of sampling and of measuring lung function.

Schoolchildren, in contrast, have been frequently used in epidemiological studies (14–17) because, where education is compulsory, all children in a given area will attend school. The population to be sampled can be easily defined from class lists and, for cohort studies, the children can be followed from year to year, often in the same schools.

Cohorts of children are particularly advantageous when studying respiratory disease and air pollution. Under the age of nine years they are unlikely to smoke cigarettes regularly (18, 19), they have no serious exposure to occupational pollutants, they tend to have a stable residential history, and their respiratory systems seem to be more sensitive to insult than those of adults, making it easier to detect adverse effects (20). Moreover, in the school years, children can carry out spirometric lung function tests satisfactorily from about seven years of age and can manage the single measurement of peak expiratory flow rate at five years of age. By the age of nine or ten years children can answer questionnaires with the help of the teacher, a technique used to obtain information on such topics as smoking habits (21) and fuel used for cooking in the home (22). Parents are usually very willing to answer questionnaires about their children's past and present health and to give information about the family and home circumstances.

In the absence of routinely collected and accessible information for schoolchildren, data must be collected by study personnel. Information from school health examinations may be suitable, but it should be collected in a standardized way (with checks for observer and machine biases when possible) so as to ensure the validity of the conclusions drawn from the results. Records of absenteeism are of limited use, unless the cause of absence can be obtained from an official source such as a general practitioner, or from hospital admission or discharge records. Causes of absence must be coarsely classified because of the non-standard way in which finer gradings of respiratory diagnosis are made, even by highly trained practitioners. On the other hand, frequency or duration of absenteeism may be useful as a measure of comparability between respondents and non-respondents.

Adults are in general not so easily enumerated as schoolchildren, except at the time of a government census. Various population lists may be available, such as lists of people and their personal numbers or electoral rolls, or it may be necessary, in the absence of any other lists, to make a private census for the purposes of a survey. Samples of adults should be used to determine the natural history of respiratory disease from its first clinical manifestations to death (*12, 23, 24*) or in situations, as in certain occupations, where only adults are liable to be exposed. Routinely collected statistics are more varied for adults than for children, and may be suitable for detecting clinical events in the study sample. Mortality data give evidence of a clear-cut end point, although the exact diagnosis may need to be confirmed, if it is required. Hospital admissions and discharges may also be used. If the study is concerned only with aggregate data (such as mortality rates for a defined population) rather than with the causes of death for specific individuals, suitable data may be obtained from local or national studies of morbidity or from registers of notifiable or prescribed diseases.

Three other groupings might be considered, the first being occupational. A population of adults can be defined by the industry in which they work, and subgroups may be formed by specific occupations within the industry. This approach is valuable if the population is stable, so that loss to the study will be small over the years, and may have particular advantages if good records of health and retirement are available. The major disadvantage that limits the generalizability of results is that the population is not representative of the general population because of self-selection and recruitment criteria.

The second grouping of adults is of those at high risk of increased severity of symptoms or disease. Asthmatics, chronic bronchitics and people with recurrent lower respiratory illness are all at increased risk of severe reactions to environmental stimuli. These reactions can be used to assess or monitor the effects of air pollutants (*25, 26*). Samples from these groups should be representative if the natural history of the disease in the clinical phases is to be studied or the results related back to the whole group.

The third grouping is suitable for genetic studies, and consists of families, parents and offspring, siblings, twins, adopted siblings and spouse pairs. It is advisable to use as many of these groups as possible in a study as none will give a definitive answer by itself.

Various populations have been described together with their attributes. Clearly, the choice will depend essentially on the question being asked, but a number of factors should be considered in the choice of a group within a given population type. Maintenance of a high response rate throughout its duration is essential to the true cohort study. Thus a stable and cooperative population is needed. Follow-up is also simplified if there is some routinely maintained register of the population, such as a register for medical practitioners or employee registers in industry. Follow-up can be improved if records are kept of the population—deaths may be found from centrally registered death certificates, or retirement histories may be obtained in industrial settings. Finally, the cohort must be young enough at the start of the study for the majority to be still available for examination at the end (unless, of course, mortality is the outcome of interest). These desirable qualities of a population are infrequently found in free living groups, but may be possessed by certain occupational groups (doctors, telephone workers, members of religious orders, etc.). If the choice of such a group seems appropriate, the consequent limited applicability or relevance of the results must be considered before a final decision is made.

SAMPLE SIZE

Once the group to be studied has been defined the question arises of how large a sample will be required. For any statistical testing of the data, more precise estimates will be obtained with increasing size of sample. However, a large sample will cost more and take longer to examine and may, through its very size, lead to errors in data collection and processing that would be avoided with a smaller, more easily comprehended sample. A balance must be found between the cost of the study, the precision of the results, and the likely value of the findings, if these can be expressed in economic terms.

In the following paragraphs the rationale for estimating the appropriate size for a sample is described. By the use of formulae, the epidemiologist can quickly decide whether the size of sample that he knows he can afford, or that is available to him, will be large enough to provide the necessary degree of precision. Alternatively, he will know whether he can reduce the size of the sample that he first postulated as adequate and still obtain the precision required to give a clear-cut answer.

The appropriate size of the sample to be drawn from a chosen population can be estimated, provided that it is clear what the expected results will be if the hypothesis to be tested is true. The formulae used to calculate sample size are derived from the tests for comparing the mean values or proportions for two groups. Where continuously distributed variables such as peak expiratory flow rate (PEFR) or vital capacity are to be compared, the t-test is the basis of the calculation. If the variables are measured as proportions, such as the proportion of people with cough first thing in the morning, then the chi-square test is the basis of the calculation.

For continuous variables, the likely mean values for both groups in the comparison must be known. The expected mean PEFR might be 560 litres/min in a normal adult group. A 5% reduction in the mean would be considered a biologically significant difference in a comparison group of smokers. Further, the probable standard deviation of the measurement must be known. For commonly measured and reported variables, it may only be necessary to look at published studies to obtain guidelines for these values. If the measurement has never been made in a similar population, a pilot study will be needed to gain an idea of the values.

The t-test is used to find the probability of an observed difference between two mean values, and is based on the assumption that the two samples concerned were drawn from the *same* population. Under these conditions, if a large number of differences are calculated from pairs of samples, the average difference (taking the sign into account) will be zero but there will be some variation about this average that would be expected to show an approximately normal distribution (Fig. 1).

In a two-tailed test the null hypothesis that the two samples in a pair were drawn from the same population is accepted if the value of the difference lies between the two hatched areas, but is rejected if the value lies in the hatched areas (the curve meets the axis only at infinity in either direction). It is obvious that the null hypothesis, although correct, may be rejected when a difference is observed that would only occur rarely. This error is known as Type I or α error. In the diagram the null hypothesis will be rejected inappropriately if the observed difference falls in the hatched areas. It is conventional for these hatched areas to account for either 5% or 1% of the total area under the distribution curve, the chosen area being divided equally between the tails in two-tailed tests or all at one end in one-tailed tests (the use of one-tailed tests is usually inappropriate). If $\alpha = 5\%$ then, as shown in Fig. 1A, $\frac{1}{2}\alpha$, or 2.5%, of the distribution lies in each hatched area. The size of α must be specified before the sample size can be calculated.

Another error is known as the Type II or β error. If the samples are drawn from two populations that are different with respect to the mean value of the variable of interest, then the average *difference* in mean values between pairs of samples will not be zero but some other value, say δ. If a large number of pairs of samples are drawn, one sample from one population and the other sample from the second population, then the differences between their means (taking the sign of the difference into account) will be distributed around δ in the way shown in Fig. 1B.

Fig. 1C shows the two distributions just described on the same axes with a degree of overlap between them. The vertical broken line marks the boundary to the right of which lies 2.5% ($\frac{1}{2}\alpha$ in this example) of the distribution of differences obtained from pairs of samples drawn from the same population. If we suppose that the difference between the means has been standardized by dividing it by its standard error, this point is 1.96 standard units above the true mean of zero. If a

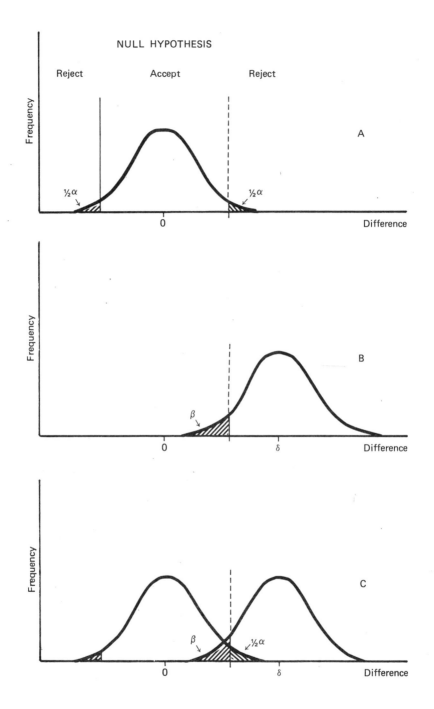

Fig. 1. Frequency distributions showing areas under the curve associated with α and β errors (see text).

standardized difference is observed that is either $\geqslant 1.96$ or $\leqslant -1.96$ (taking both tails into account) the null hypothesis will be rejected with a 5% chance that a Type I error has been made.

Most of the distribution with mean δ lies to the right of the vertical dashed line so that, if δ were the true difference, a large proportion of possible sample values for the differences in means between two differing populations would appropriately lie in the area of rejection of the null hypothesis. The left-hand tail of the distribution, however, lies in the area where the null hypothesis would be inappropriately accepted (Type II error). The amount of overlap can be specified beforehand; typical percentages (β) of the distribution centred about δ that are used are 5, 10 or 20%. This means that 5, 10 or 20 out of 100 sample differences taken at random would have values so close to zero that the null hypothesis would be accepted, when in fact it should be rejected. If the β error is chosen as 10%, the standardized distance from δ to the vertical line in Fig. 1C is 1.28. The point on the abscissa so defined is the same as that obtained in the α error calculations, thus:

$$0.0 + 1.96\text{SE} = \delta - 1.28\text{SE}$$

or
$$1.96 = \delta/\text{SE} - 1.28 \tag{1}$$

where SE is the standard error of the difference.

For the calculation of sample size, the population variances that are estimated from the two samples are assumed to be equal. The estimated pooled variance (S^2) is an average of the two estimated variances from the samples, each weighted by the number of observations used in its calculation. The standard error of the difference between the means of the samples is:

$$\sqrt{\frac{S^2}{n_1} + \frac{S^2}{n_2}}$$

For a given value of $(n_1 + n_2)$ the smallest standard error is obtained when $n_1 = n_2 = n$, thus:

$$\text{SE} = \sqrt{\frac{2S^2}{n}}$$

Equation (1) then becomes:

$$1.96 = \frac{\delta}{\sqrt{\dfrac{2S^2}{n}}} - 1.28$$

Hence
$$\delta^2 = (1.96 + 1.28)^2 \cdot 2 \frac{S^2}{n}$$

and
$$n = 2 \left[(1.96 + 1.28) \frac{S}{\delta} \right]^2 \tag{2}$$

where n is the size of *each* group (i.e. total sample size is $2n$ for 2 groups).

Equation (2) can be generalized by using $Z_{(100-\alpha)}$ to indicate the boundary on the normal distribution for one-tailed tests or $Z_{(100-\frac{1}{2}\alpha)}$ for

25

two-tailed tests, while $Z_{(100-\beta)}$ indicates the β boundary on the standard normal distribution. Thus equation (2) becomes:

$$n = 2\left[(Z_{(100-\frac{1}{2}\alpha)} + Z_{(100-\beta)})\frac{S}{\delta}\right]^2 \tag{3}$$

To calculate the number of observations necessary, values are needed for all the symbols on the right of the equals sign—levels for α and β and their corresponding points on the standard normal distribution, the probable standard deviation of the individuals' observations (S in the formula), and the true difference between the two sample means that is thought to be biologically important.

In cohort studies, if the observations are made on the same individual at two separate times, or on matched pairs of exposed and unexposed individuals, the equation becomes:

$$n = \left[(Z_{(100-\frac{1}{2}\alpha)} + Z_{(100-\beta)})\frac{S}{\delta}\right]^2 \tag{4}$$

where n is now the number of paired observations and S^2 is the variance of the differences between the pairs.

If proportions or rates are to be compared (e.g. the proportion of people with asthma), the equations for n look somewhat different, although the same basic concepts underlie them. A two-step procedure is used to calculate n, as follows:

$$n' = \frac{(Z_{(100-\frac{1}{2}\alpha)}\sqrt{(2\overline{P}\,\overline{Q})} + Z_{(100-\beta)}\sqrt{(p_1 q_1 + p_2 q_2)})^2}{\delta^2} \tag{5}$$

where $\overline{P} = (p_1 + p_2)/2$, $\overline{Q} = (1 - \overline{P})$, p_1 and p_2 are the expected proportions in the two samples, and $q_i = (1 - p_i)$ (27).

Then (28)
$$n = \frac{n'}{4}\left[1 + \sqrt{\left(1 + \frac{4}{n'\delta}\right)}\right]^2 \tag{6}$$

The rather cumbersome equation for n' can be replaced by the following equation from Cochran & Cox (29), which gives almost the same results and is simpler to work out with a hand-held calculator:

$$n' = (Z_{(100-\frac{1}{2}\alpha)} + Z_{(100-\beta)})^2 / [2(\sin^{-1}\sqrt{p_1} - \sin^{-1}\sqrt{p_2})^2] \tag{7}$$

where $\sqrt{p_i}$ is considered to be in radians.
Two examples show how equations (3), (6) and (7) are used.

Example 1

It has been found that the mean value for PEFR in a group of normal adults is 560 litres/min. Mean PEFR in a group exposed to an atmospheric pollutant is considered to have been reduced to a biologically significant degree if it is 5% lower than normal (i.e. 532 litres/min), so that $\delta = 28$ litres/min. The standard deviation (SD) of PEFR is 30 litres/min. A two-tailed test will be used (because it is possible that the exposed group may have an elevated PEFR) and the value of α is set at 5%. A 90% chance of finding a difference if one really exists is required (i.e. $\beta = 10\%$). What sample size is necessary?

By reference to tables of the standard normal distribution:

$$Z_{(100-\frac{1}{2}\alpha)} = 1.96$$

$$Z_{(100-\beta)} = 1.28$$

$$SD = 30$$

$$\delta = 28.$$

Then, from equation (3):

$$n = 24.$$

Example 2

The proportion with cough first thing in the morning in a normal adult population of males has been found to be 15%. If this proportion were 25% in a group exposed to an atmospheric pollutant, the increase would be considered of biological importance. If α is set at 1%, a two-tailed test is used, and β is set at 5%, we have:

$$Z_{(100-\frac{1}{2}\alpha)} = 2.58$$

$$Z_{(100-\beta)} = 1.645$$

$$p_1 = 0.15$$

$$p_2 = 0.25$$

Then, from equations (6) and (7) we obtain:

$$n = 583.$$

The calculation of n is complex for studies in which observations are made on more than two occasions; it will depend on the statistical methods to be used at the completion of the fieldwork and requires the services of a competent statistician.

SAMPLING

When the sample size has been estimated, the way the sample is to be selected must be chosen. The purpose of the sampling procedure is to obtain a group of people who are representative of a defined larger population to which the results of the study are to be applied.

If the selection of the sample is left to the discretion of the investigator it is unlikely that it will have characteristics similar to those of the population from which it was drawn (i.e. it will not be representative). This is because there will be both intentional and unintentional biases imposed on the selection, such as obtaining people from convenient locations (intentional) and failure to appreciate the need to follow up non-respondents (unintentional). These biases may be

27

avoided by using sampling methods that do not depend on decisions made by the investigator.

A number of methods for choosing samples are available,[a] of which three will be considered here.

Systematic sampling

The population from which the sample is to be drawn may be listed or may, for example, be a file of medical records in a fixed order and of known number. The sampling fraction is calculated from the ratio n/N, where n is the sample size and N is the size of the population. If we need a sample of 100 people from a list of 9000, the sampling fraction would be 100/9000 or 1 in 90. To obtain the 100 people by systematic sampling, every 90th person would be selected. The first person selected should be chosen at random from the first 90 people on the list or the first 90 records in the file; this random selection could be made by reference to a set of random number tables. The sample is made up of the first record plus all following records at intervals of 90 records. This method works well provided that there are no cyclical changes in the list of people corresponding to the frequency of the sampling fraction. For instance, if every 90th person in our example was a manager in an industry but the remainder were shop floor workers, the sample would not be representative of the total since it would perforce include only managers or only workers. Evidence should be obtained that this is not the case for a particular list and sampling fraction; this might be done by comparing two samples starting at different randomly selected points, each at half the sampling rate (e.g. 1 in 180). If they are similar they can be combined to form the required sample.

Random sampling

Systematic sampling is subject to biases that may not be easy to detect. They may be avoided by random sampling, in which the probability of selection into the sample is the same for all individuals. Two types of random sample are considered here: the simple random sample, where everyone in the population has an equal chance of selection; and the stratified random sample, in which the population is divided into groups (strata) according to one or more characteristics, and everyone in each group has the same probability of selection but the probability differs from one stratum to another.

If every member of the population has been identified, usually by means of some kind of census, a simple random sample can be taken. Each member is given a number. As many random numbers are obtained

---

[a] For more detailed information, any of the excellent books on sampling methods should be consulted. The aim here is merely to draw the reader's attention to the importance of avoiding bias in the selection of a sample and the means of achieving this.

from a table as are required for the sample and these are matched with the names on the list. These selected people form the sample.

The stratified random sample is one in which simple random samples are taken from defined groups within the total population, each at a different sampling fraction. In this way those groups that might have had few people in them if only a simple random sample from the total population had been taken (such as people aged over 80) can be increased in size so that they can be analysed separately without loss of randomness of selection. This procedure also allows a more precise estimate of population parameters by ensuring that small groups in the population with outlying characteristics are included in every sample.

An example of the use of stratified sampling is given by Fletcher et al. (*12*). They chose two stable populations of males in the United Kingdom, one in the London Transport workshops and the other in the Post Office Savings Bank. A small preliminary questionnaire survey was made to establish whether the prevalence of bronchitic symptoms was high enough to justify a long-term study. This was followed by a questionnaire to all men (3013) aged 30–59 years to identify those who had symptoms, so that a sample of 1000 men stratified by symptoms could be drawn for follow-up. Four strata were defined: symptomatic men (including those on sick leave for respiratory illness), asymptomatic non-smokers, asymptomatic smokers or ex-smokers and, finally, those who did not return the questionnaire but who were willing to take part in the survey. Sampling fractions for these groups were 100%, 50%, 20% and 30%, respectively. This scheme was used so that all men with symptoms could be followed, the proportion of non-smokers would be greater than that in the whole group, and the proportion of the many asymptomatic smokers would be reduced. Although this particular stratification scheme has obvious advantages, the authors pointed out that stratification based on only one factor (smoking) would have greatly simplified the analyses.

CHAPTER 3

Examination techniques

The two previous chapters have outlined the general methodology of cohort studies and the types of population that can be investigated. In this chapter, methods for measuring relevant personal characteristics of these populations are discussed. Many of these measurements will be made in the same way whatever the final form of the cohort study and the hypothesis to be tested, and are therefore described in some detail.

The use of well-tried instruments and measurements is emphasized because of their acceptance by many workers. Much is known about their validity and reliability. The choice of methods has also been based on a number of considerations other than familiarity. The instrument should be easily portable (e.g. a peak expiratory flow meter or a questionnaire) so that it can be carried from house to house if necessary. It should be possible to make the measurement rapidly so that the time a respondent spends being examined can be kept acceptably short; this includes the questionnaire, which should be brief enough to ensure that all the questions are read and answered. Lung function instruments should be easily calibrated in the field and should be capable of standardization so that bias is not introduced into the results because of variability in the machines themselves.

This chapter is divided into two main sections dealing with standard questionnaires and with lung function tests respectively; special investigations, such as chest radiography, are also included. The text is concerned solely with the measurement of the human respondent and his surroundings as he perceives them. This may give the impression that it is these measurements to which most attention must be devoted during the planning stage of a project, particularly since the hypothesis to be tested is likely to be concerned with human health. However, in studies of the effects of air pollutants on the respiratory system, the measurement of the pollutant is equally important; the method, its validity and reliability and the biases affecting it must be thoroughly understood. Often the epidemiologist will not be competent in such measurement, and it is not the intention here to attempt to describe any of the methods for measuring the multiplicity of possible pollutants. This lack of emphasis on a critical aspect of environmental studies is not, however, to deny the importance of sound measurement of the environment. It is very easy for health-oriented epidemiologists planning a study either to accept uncritically whatever environmental measurements happen to be made in the study area or to postpone consideration of the measurements until the health aspects of the protocol have been completed. These attitudes must be avoided at all costs; the environmental measures must be included in the plans from the start and their suitability for the study tested in as exacting a way as are the measures of health status. It is essential, therefore, to have an environmental expert as a member of the planning group.

THE QUESTIONNAIRE

Information on individuals is usually collected directly, rather than from records. This makes it possible to obtain in a standardized way answers to all the questions that the investigator thinks are relevant. Questionnaires have been part of the respiratory epidemiologist's equipment for many years because they offer the only way in which a history of symptoms can be obtained. Three standard questionnaires have been developed: one by the British Medical Research Council (MRC) during the 1950s, which was designed for the investigation of the natural history of chronic bronchitis; one by the United States National Heart and Lung Institute (NHLI), which was a modification of the MRC questionnaire for use in the USA; and one by the American Thoracic Society (ATS), which was based on the MRC questionnaire but was expanded to allow investigation of a wider range of problems.

All three questionnaires contain questions on certain core items of information. The information needed to identify the respondent includes the name and address, which are linked to a unique survey number. Where confidentiality of the data must be assured, the identification data should be collected on separate forms that can only be linked to the questionnaire by the study number. These forms and the questionnaires can be kept separately; the forms will be needed to identify respondents for follow-up examinations. Many countries will have national guidelines for preserving confidentiality in health studies.

Other basic data include identification of the interviewers, if they are used, for analysis of interviewer bias so that corrections to the results may be included in the findings. The date of interview and the respondent's date of birth must be included so that age can be calculated accurately. It is not sufficient to ask the respondent's age directly as there is a tendency in some groups to deny entering a new decade or in others to exaggerate their age. The age need not be calculated by the interviewer if the data are later to be processed by computer, but it is wise to make a rough calculation to guard against obvious errors at a time when they can be easily corrected with the respondent's help. Sex, race, marital status and place of birth are also required as they may be related to the frequency of symptoms or the level of lung function. If the respondent is a schoolchild, the school's name or code should be noted.

These questions designed to obtain basic demographic data are followed by questions on respiratory symptoms and past illness. The position of these questions is very important as the answers should not be influenced by the respondent's reaction to other questions, particularly on smoking habits or occupation, both of which are generally known to affect the respiratory system. Questions on occupation or smoking must follow those on symptoms but their own order is less critical. Information on family history of respiratory disease may also be sought. If any other questions need to be added to a standard questionnaire, they must be placed at the end so that they will not influence the answers to the standard questions.

The questionnaire must be designed so that the results can be coded for data processing. This is not an unskilled task; it should be done by someone with experience. Many mistakes have been made by investigators unfamiliar with computing practice who have considered the job to be too trivial for outside help to be needed.

When a questionnaire has been written it should be tested for reliability and validity. Reliability refers to the ability of the questionnaire to elicit the same answers on two or more occasions, validity to the ability of the questionnaire to measure what was intended. The repeatability of questionnaire data can be measured by "consistency" or the κ statistic, and the validity by sensitivity and specificity. The method of calculating these statistics is given in Annex 1. The questionnaire should also be evaluated for observer bias if it is to be administered by interviewers.

THE STANDARD QUESTIONNAIRES

The use of standard questionnaires avoids the problems raised in the previous paragraphs and makes comparison of results between studies more reliable. In cooperative studies they are essential.

The MRC questionnaire

The MRC questionnaire was conceived in the 1950s, first published in 1960, and revised in 1966 and 1976. Annex 2 gives the latest revision and includes the instructions for its use.

This questionnaire, in its original version, was evaluated in postal workers in some detail (30, 31). Answers to questions about the amount of phlegm produced each day correlated well with morning sputum volume, and the expected relations existed between grade of phlegm and prevalence of symptoms and indirect maximal breathing capacity.

Answers to questions on chest illness correlated reasonably well with work sickness records in men but not in women; under- and over-reporting were of about equal frequency in men. Other authors have found similar results. The answers to the questionnaire have been compared with clinical diagnoses. A reasonably close relation between the two was found in the United Kingdom, but the relation was weaker in a study in the United States.

Validation of the MRC questionnaire has been based principally on the relation between reported and observed phlegm production. The other symptom questions have not been validated because of the lack of an independent criterion, but have been found to be associated with reduced forced expiratory volume in 1 second (FEV_1).

The reliability of the questionnaire has been measured by administering it on two occasions fairly close together in time to the same group of people, to determine whether there was any change in the answers. The consistency of the questions on phlegm was between 75 % and 90 % in the United Kingdom (*30, 32*) and the Netherlands (*33*) but rather less in the United States (*34*). The questions on smoking status were very reliable (99 %) in the United Kingdom and calculated lifetime cigarette consumption showed good correlation (0.8) between interviews in a study in the United States.

The results obtained from questionnaires may be biased by effects introduced by interviewers, the method of administration, questionnaire modification and seasonal effects.

The answers interviewers obtain depend on the way in which the questions are put. Both departure from the printed wording and non-verbal clues as to how the interviewer would like the respondent to answer will influence the results. This bias may be measured by having two interviewers administer the questionnaire to the same people. In order to separate the learning effect from the interviewer bias, the order of the interviewers (first or second) should be varied. Another possibility is for each interviewer to question a random sample of a group of people in the expectation that the results should be the same, allowing for sampling error. Neither method is completely satisfactory, but they can give some insight into the errors introduced by interviewers.

Early studies, in which the second method was used, showed that interviewer bias could be substantial and even lead to a doubling of the prevalence of some symptoms. Subsequently, during the development of the MRC questionnaire, detailed printed instructions for the interviewers were prepared. These explained the meaning of such words as "usually" and described how probing should be done for those questions where it was allowed. Early results (*30, 31*) of experiments on bias, where a mixture of the two approaches described above was used and the interviews were recorded on tape, showed that 62 % of the errors were made by the interviewers, 21 % were made by the subjects, and 16 % were due to the wording of the question. This led to the rewording of some of the questions and a realization of the importance of training the interviewers in the details of the instructions, since most of the interviewer errors were due to failure to follow the rules. Subsequent tests of interviewer bias (*32, 35*), when the MRC questionnaire and properly trained interviewers were used, showed minimal or no significant effects.

Questionnaires may be administered by interviewer or be self-administered. The latter method avoids the biases introduced by an intermediary and is much cheaper. Difficulties arise from self-administered questionnaires when the respondent fails to answer all the questions or fails to return the questionnaire to the researcher, or when someone else other than the intended respondent completes the questionnaire. To reduce non-response, the language and the instructions must be readily understood by the respondent and the structure of the questionnaire should be attractive and easy to follow, particularly where there are branching questions. Other difficulties may arise in cohort studies from a training effect on the respondent after repeated use of the questionnaire, though this is probably not very marked (*12*), and from the general public's attitude towards the subject under study. Samet et al. (*34*) found a 50 % increase in major symptoms in asbestos workers over one year, when the hazards of asbestos had become general knowledge, although neither pulmonary function nor chest radiographs showed any change.

The MRC questionnaire was originally designed for interviewer administration but has been adapted for self-administration. Comparison of results using both methods showed a consistency of 85 % for the questions on chronic cough and phlegm (*36*). The same level of agreement was found in the United States in a comparison between interview responses from the MRC questionnaire and responses from self-administration of the NHLI questionnaire, which has similarly worded questions (*34*).

Modification of the questionnaire may give rise to considerable differences in response. Holland et al. (*32*) compared the results of the Pneumoconiosis Field Research (PFR) and the MRC questionnaires on the same group of coal miners. The PFR questionnaire was specifically designed to ask for one item of information in each question, whereas the MRC questionnaire contained questions where multiple conditions had to be satisfied before a positive answer could be given (see for example Annex 2, question 1). Although the two questionnaires were seeking the same information, the different styles led to substantial differences in the estimates of prevalence of symptoms and chronic bronchitis. Thus, if a standardized questionnaire is to be used and the results are to be as comparable as possible with other studies, no question should be modified. If any question is modified, the change must be described so that others working in the field may judge what effects the change may have on results.

Bias may be introduced when results from the questionnaire used at two different times of the year are compared. Questions referring to symptoms occurring during the winter might be expected to have higher positive responses if asked in the winter or spring than in the other seasons, because the symptoms will be more readily remembered. However, in several studies (*30, 32, 33*) this bias has not been consistently found. Because it may occur, however, it is wise either to have follow-up examinations at the same time each year or to design the study so that any bias that does arise can be detected.

The MRC questionnaire, when used properly, is not biased by the interviewers, the mode of administration and probably not by the season. It has been translated into many languages and has been in use now for over 20 years. For studies on adults, it is the questionnaire of choice as it is well tested, its characteristics are known and results can be compared with those from the many other studies in which it has been used.

The NHLI and ATS-DLD-78 questionnaires

The two standard American questionnaires were derived from the MRC questionnaire but have been adapted to make them more suitable for use in the United States, and to increase the information obtained in particular areas.

The NHLI questionnaire was released in 1971 in response to the needs of investigators for broader enquiries than provided by the MRC questionnaire. The NHLI and MRC questionnaires were not compared at that time. In 1974 the American Thoracic Society (ATS), under contract to the Division of Lung Diseases (DLD) of the National Heart, Lung and Blood Institute, began developing a questionnaire specifically for use in epidemiological studies. This made use of questions already contained in the MRC and NHLI questionnaires and added detailed questions, particularly on asthma, smoking history and history of family health.

All three questionnaires were assessed in a single study in a general population in Washington County, Maryland (*37*). The method was to administer the three questionnaires over the telephone or to send them by mail (6 possibilities) to six groups of 200 white people aged 25–64 years, each with similar distributions by sex, age, education, cigarette smoking and area of residence within the county. All respondents to the interview and all people sent the mailed questionnaire were invited to undergo lung function tests at a central site. Two interviewers and four part-time spirometer technicians collected the data.

Table 4 shows some of the results of comparisons between the three questionnaires. The NHLI questionnaire, although obtaining similar results to the other questionnaires for some symptoms, diverged substantially for others, whereas the MRC and ATS-DLD questionnaires gave similar results throughout (with the exception of the question "any wheeze"). All three questionnaires had similar sensitivity, as shown by the prevalence of symptoms that increased at similar rates with increases in cigarette smoking and decreases in FEV_1. The variation in responses according to the method of administration was not significant for the MRC or ATS-DLD questionnaires, but the symptom of breathlessness

Table 4. Percentage of respondents with respiratory symptoms elicited by three questionnaires used in Washington County, MD, USA(*37*)

Symptom	Percentage reporting symptom		
	MRC	NHLI	ATS – DLD
Chronic cough	29.4	21.4	22.0
Chronic phlegm	21.7	23.1	20.2
Any wheeze	31.5	37.4	51.9[a]
Moderate breathlessness	34.1	46.9[a]	34.8
Severe breathlessness	11.6	16.9	14.6
Recent chest illness	11.3	43.9[a]	15.2
Chronic wheeze	12.4	–	14.8
Asthma	5.6	–	4.8
Hay fever	14.5	–	12.0

[a] $P < 0.01$ for difference between this percentage and the other percentages in the same row.

was significantly more frequently reported in the mailed compared with the interviewer-administered NHLI questionnaires. Comparability among interviewers was unconditionally good for the MRC, good for the ATS-DLD (with the exception of the question on breathlessness) but substantially worse for the NHLI questionnaire, for which there were significant differences between interviewers for answers to the questions on chronic phlegm and breathlessness.

The percentage of questions not answered or with incomprehensible responses in the mailed questionnaires was nearly 7% for the MRC questionnaire, compared with about $4\frac{1}{4}$% for the other questionnaires.

In another study in Washington County, the MRC and ATS-DLD questionnaires were both given to 946 white males, half of whom received the MRC questionnaire first (*38*). No important differences attributable to the order of administration were found. Both found similar proportions of respondents with cough, phlegm, wheeze, breathlessness and chest illness in the previous three years (though not for previous illness lasting one week or more), so that they both gave comparable estimates of the prevalence of chronic bronchitis.

Of the two United States questionnaires, the ATS-DLD-78 (Annex 3) is recommended. It has been extensively investigated, and the symptom and past illness questions have been found to be repeatable, valid and to give results for the most part similar to those obtained from the MRC questionnaire. It has the advantage of containing more detailed questions than the latter.

For studies of adults, the choice of questionnaire will depend on the problem under investigation, on the need for comparability with previous studies, on availability in the appropriate languages and, in cooperative studies, on the complete agreement of all principal investigators.

The history and testing of respiratory symptoms questionnaires has been reviewed by Samet (39).

CHILDREN'S QUESTIONNAIRES

Questionnaires for children have been used for some time but none has been standardized or adequately assessed for reliability or validity. Two questionnaires have been widely used in Europe, one prepared by WHO (40) and the other by the Directorate-General for Research, Science and Education of the Commission of the European Communities (the CEC questionnaire). Both have been used in cooperative studies started in the 1970s and have proved acceptable to respondents when given by interview. An extensive (unpublished) analysis of the relation between symptoms obtained from the CEC questionnaire and PEFR indicated that many of the symptoms were associated with lower PEFR levels but that the extent varied from one country to another. The most consistent relation was found between PEFR and the presence of at least one symptom of respiratory illness in the last 12 months (any positive answer to questions 1–3 and 5–8).

These two questionnaires and instructions for their use are given in Annexes 4 and 5, respectively.

A third, untested questionnaire (ATS-DLD-78-C) has been prepared by the American Thoracic Society (41).

The same considerations need to be taken into account in the choice of questionnaire as those mentioned in connection with adult questionnaires.

TRAINING OF INTERVIEWERS

Interviewers should be able to read aloud clearly and to follow instructions precisely. Physicians are rarely good interviewers for epidemiological studies because they are trained to assess responses in a non-standard way, and respondents may be more inclined to please a physician by giving the answers that they believe him to want.

Research on observer variation in interviews has made it clear that interviewers must be trained to use the questionnaire that they are to administer. *The results of a study where training has been omitted are valueless even when a standard questionnaire has been used.* It is essential, therefore, for a training programme to be included in the design of the study.

The training should consist of three steps. Tape recordings of simulated interviews should be prepared, both of correctly performed sessions and of sessions where errors are made and corrected according to the interviewer's instruction manual. Each interview should be conducted twice, a different respondent being used the second time so as to conceal this fact.

Trainees should be given time to read and consider the questionnaire (but not the instructions). They should then attempt to write down the answers on a questionnaire form on the basis of what they have understood from the tape recording. Their results should be compared with the correct answers. The untrained interviewer is very likely to make mistakes in this process, and may make different mistakes when the same interview is repeated. The point of this activity is to demonstrate to the trainees the need for training to eliminate errors. It provides the motivation to succeed.

The trainees should then be introduced to the written instructions for the questionnaire and should be given time to understand them and learn them by heart. They should practise, using each other as respondents, to become familiar with the flow of questions. They should then repeat the exercise with the first tape recording to see how they have improved, and again with a recording of different interviews that bring out all the problems that the instructions were designed to eliminate. The results should be discussed in a group session with the trainers.

Those trainees who show no aptitude for interviewing might be dropped from the course at this stage. The remainder should use the questionnaire with volunteer respondents to gain experience of live interviews. These interviews should be recorded (with the respondents' permission) for later review by the trainers and trainees.

This whole process may take up to a week before interviewers are ready to conduct independent interviews. In studies in which several interviewers are used, respondents should be randomly assigned to the interviewers and each interviewer should be identified on the questionnaire. In this way an assessment of inter-observer bias can be made at the end of the survey.

ADDITIONAL QUESTIONS

If questions are to be added to a standard questionnaire, they should be placed at the end so that the answers to the original questions will not be contaminated by them and comparability will be retained with other studies in which the same questionnaire is used.

New questions must be carefully worded and tested on people similar to those to whom the questionnaire will be administered in the main study. The answers should be suitable for computer analysis, and the design of the questionnaire should make both the coding and the transfer to machine-readable form as simple as possible. For the design of questionnaires for epidemiological studies, see Bennett & Ritchie (42).

DIARIES

If changes in symptoms or in feeling of well-being are of interest, they may be recorded in a diary. This technique has been used to follow the experience of chronic bronchitics as pollution levels in London varied from day to day (25). Each patient was given a thin booklet that could fit easily into a small pocket. Instructions for its use were printed inside the cover. Patients were asked to record whether they felt better, the same or worse than the day before. These responses were coded 1, 2 and 3, respectively, and the daily mean value for all patients was plotted against the daily levels of outside smoke and sulfur dioxide. In years when the pollutant levels were high on average and showed marked fluctuation, the diary score was closely related to pollutant levels, but this correlation disappeared in the years when the levels had been brought under control.

This particular approach is very simple. The diary can always be at hand, since it can be carried in the pocket without inconvenience, and the demand on the patient is minimal, requiring the entry of only one word each day. More complex diaries may be designed, but must be assessed for ease of completion, the respondent's compliance in making regular entries, and the length of time that respondents are willing to continue making entries. They will be suitable only for literate populations.

LUNG FUNCTION MEASUREMENTS

In recent years there has been a growing understanding of the nature of the pathology of various forms of serious lung disease. At the same time there has been a trend towards greater emphasis on the use of pulmonary function measurements in epidemiological studies, as functional abnormalities seem to be of key importance in lowering the quality of life.

Most epidemiological studies seek to find evidence of airway obstruction from measurements of expiratory flow rates and timed expiratory volumes, and particularly from the forced expiratory volume in 1 second (FEV_1). Recently, tests considered to be more sensitive to minor degrees of airway obstruction, such as flow rates in the second half of forced maximal expiration, have come into vogue. The choice of a lung function test should be made in consultation with a respiratory physiologist, but it should not be forgotten that the best test in any situation is the one that meets the requirements of portability, rapid performance, reliability and capacity for standardization in the field, and yet measures the functional attributes appropriate to the objective of the study.

Furthermore, high sensitivity does not necessarily confer an unqualified advantage on a test from the point of view of its use in an epidemiological survey. Frequently, the more sensitive the test, the greater the variation among individuals and therefore the larger the sample needed to detect a given change. Thus in determining which pulmonary function test to use, not only must a decision first be made as to what characteristic of the lung is to be examined in detail, but the characteristics of the proposed test, and particularly its natural variance, need to be taken into account. Many of the difficulties with pulmonary function tests in epidemiological studies arise because the tests have been developed within the clinical setting. When the patient with established lung disease is to be assessed, or when fairly gross diagnoses are to be made, variations between machines or small observer errors are unimportant. However, when these same sources of error occur in the epidemiological setting, disaster can follow. Differences in lung function of a fairly minor degree between two populations can be wrongly imputed to exposure to some factor, whereas they are completely attributable, in reality, to variations between the machines or observers used in measuring lung function in the two populations. This has been found in studies using the Wright peak expiratory flow meter, which is notoriously difficult to standardize and calibrate. Such an instrument, where the observer has to read from a scale, introduces all the errors of digit preference and observer variation that have consistently plagued surveys of blood pressure.

The following questions should therefore be asked in choosing a test for use in an epidemiological survey.

1. What aspect of lung function is to be examined—airway obstruction, lung restriction, diminished lung volume, minor changes in later expiratory flow rate, or some other factor, such as bronchial reactivity?

2. Are fairly gross changes in lung function or only subtle changes to be used in determining whether a population is at risk of developing serious functional abnormality?

3. What is the range of physiological techniques for the measurement of this variable?

4. What differences between the exposed and unexposed populations are expected in this variable?

5. What is the natural variation in the measurement and, consequently, what size of sample will be required to detect, with stated certainty, differences of biological interest?

6. How far does the suggested technique meet the requirements of portability, speed, reliability and easy standardization in the field?

An extensive review by the American Thoracic Society (ATS) of lung function tests suitable for epidemiological studies (*41*) contains a very detailed examination of numerous procedures, and of the equipment required for their execution. An attempt is made to use established knowledge as a basis for recommendations as to procedures, apparatus, measurements and calibration for various tests and for identifying areas where further research is necessary in evaluating the usefulness and appropriateness of a particular test. Some of the more important aspects of the review are summarized below, but the reader is referred to the original publication for details of apparatus, procedure, rationale and relevant literature references.

Spirometry

The forced vital capacity (FVC) and the forced respiratory volume in 1 second are "the simplest, most repeatable, valid, and among the more discriminating tests reflecting mechanics and breathing. They have had most extensive trials during the past 25 years, and regression equations for predicted normal performance are better documented than for any other respiratory test" (*41*). The ATS recommendation was that these two tests should be an integral part of all respiratory epidemiological studies.

An extensive range of apparatus is currently available for recording these variables, including:

    (*a*) non-counter-weighted water spirometers;

    (*b*) rolling-seal spirometers;

    (*c*) wedge spirometers; and

    (*d*) electronic devices that measure respiratory flow throughout a forced maximal expiration, and then integrate it with time to determine volume.

All equipment must be assessed carefully before it is used in field surveys. Obvious requirements, such as portability, must be satisfied. Whatever equipment is chosen, it should have a 7-litre minimum volume capacity and a 12-litre/s flow limit, so that the upper limits of almost the entire population will be covered. The equipment should have a minimal accuracy of $\pm 3\%$ of the reading or ± 0.05 litres, whichever is the greater. Most of the volume interpreting devices will satisfy this criterion although some machines, based on a pneumotachograph, may fall short. The use of this type of equipment to produce recordings that are immediately digitalized, without the production of visual "hard copy", is to be avoided. Such a system is very difficult to calibrate when contained in a single "black box" without output to check performance at the time of measurement or, later, to assist in explaining unusual results.

For comparative purposes, volumes obtained by spirometry must be corrected for other variables that may affect these measurements, including age, sex, race, standing height, barometric pressure and temperature. The use of a nose clip is not considered mandatory and the results appear to be independent of the position in which spirometry is conducted (standing or sitting).

Adequate performance of the forced vital capacity manoeuvre requires some instruction on the subject. Often this is best achieved by demonstrating the procedure to groups of 10–20 subjects at a time. Once the subjects have shown in practice that they understand the manoeuvre, can commence briskly, apparently put all their effort into it and exhale completely, three formal recordings should be made for each individual (practice blows should be recorded; see Chapter 4). If these are performed adequately, the variation between records in the same individual should not be greater than 5%. Because the procedure depends on assessing function under circumstances of maximum effort, the largest of the three recordings is used for the final results (see Chapter 4). Corrections can then be made to this value for ambient conditions and the result given as a percentage of regression equation predictions for an individual of appropriate height, race and age. The so-called "percent predicted" values for FEV_1 or FVC are commonly quoted figures.

Frequent regular calibration of equipment for measuring spirometric variables is of crucial importance if electronic devices are involved, especially those measuring flow. Calibration of volume measuring devices is much less of a problem, although it should be carried out regularly in consultation with a pulmonary physiologist who has in his laboratory the necessary devices for that purpose. This is discussed in detail in the ATS review.

Peak expiratory flow rate (PEFR)

PEFR has been commonly measured in epidemiological surveys carried out in Europe over the past 20 years. The chief advantage of this form of test is the portability of the Wright and other peak expiratory flow meters, and the ease with which measurements can be made under the most difficult field conditions. The Wright peak expiratory flow meter requires no power source, is light in weight, and can be used with children and adults alike. However, it has not found wide favour in the United States; in fact no mention of measurement of peak expiratory flow rate alone is made in the ATS review. The test is not popular among respiratory physiologists because the measurement is based on a highly effort-dependent portion of the forced expiration curve, and also in part because no-one is clear as to what the key components of the physiological determination of the peak expiratory flow rate really are. However, they include the strength of the respiratory muscles, the calibre and compliance of the airways, and the elastic properties of the parenchyma. They also include the frequency response characteristics of the measuring device, which are critically important if different instruments are used to measure PEFR. Thus the interpretation of abnormalities in this test is difficult, if not impossible.

The most popular form of instrument in previous epidemiological studies has been the simple hand-held Wright peak expiratory flow meter. However, it is possible to obtain measurements of PEFR as incidental variables if an entire record is made of expiratory flow rates throughout a forced maximal expiration, as in some of the forms of flow measurement on which electronic spirometry or measurement of the maximal expiratory flow volume (MEFV) curve are based.

The instructions to the subject will vary, depending on the technique used to measure peak expiratory flow rate. Thus if it is being recorded as part of a measurement of expiratory flow throughout the entire forced maximal expiratory phase, the instructions will be the same as those given for spirometry (using an electronic device) or for measuring the MEFV curve. If the Wright peak expiratory flow meter is being used, or some equivalent instrument, the subject should be given a demonstration of its use. The results of five blows should be recorded (see Chapter 4).

Calibration of Wright expiratory flow meters remains a major unsolved difficulty that severely limits the usefulness of this device. One way in which some estimate of the contribution of machine variation to the measurement can be made is by asking the field workers to blow into all of their machines at the start of each day's work and to record their own PEFR as measured by the different machines. The machine number should be noted on the record of each subject so that any constant deviation attributable to a particular recording device can be taken into account in due course in the analysis of the results. Regression equations exist for peak expiratory flow, although they generally do not explain as much of the variation in peak flow as do the equations for the spirometric variables.

Other tests

A number of other tests are available for investigating specific disease states. For example, if interstitial lung disease is suspected, as may be the case in industrially exposed populations, tests measuring diffusion and other components of lung volume may be entirely appropriate. If airway obstruction is the disease of particular interest, alternatives exist to spirometry or PEFR; in particular, a number of variables can be easily measured by the flow volume loop.

Since the work by Leuallen & Fowler in 1955 (43), it has been increasingly recognized that large accelerations and decelerations of flow occur during the first few tenths of a second of forced expiration. If the mean flow rate is measured over the range 25–75% of FVC (FEF 25–75%)[a] this provides more information derived from the effort-independent section of the curve than does PEFR and is determined more by the characteristics of the airways.

---

[a] FEF: forced expiratory flow.

FEF 25–75% is determined, in physiological terms, by flow through both large- and small-diameter airways. It is thus possible for disease of the small airways to reduce FEF 25–75% in the absence of large-airways disease. However, a decrease in FEF 25–75% cannot be interpreted as specifically due to a change in small airways, although it may indicate possible small-airways abnormality if the large airways are normal. This point is of considerable significance, since chronic obstructive pulmonary disease may well have its origin in the smaller airways.

Flow rates of 25%, 50% and 75% of FVC can be measured automatically by computer from the MEFV curve or, alternatively, they can be determined manually from a "hard copy" of the MEFV loop.

The apparatus for obtaining the flow rates at 25, 50 and 75% of FVC is the same as that used for the electronic tabulation of spirometry. If a non-electronic device is used, the FEF 25–75% can be calculated manually, from a hard copy spirogram. The total FVC is measured and a line then drawn through the 25–75% volume points so as to intersect two time lines 1 second apart. This provides a measure of the number of litres per second. A much more reliable alternative to the manual determination of the FEF 25–75% is its calculation by microprocessor attached to the pulmonary function testing equipment.

It is highly controversial whether the amount of information derived from the timed expiratory volume and its various flow rates exceeds what might be obtained through the use of spirometry. Many of the flow rates described above have large variances, so that larger samples are required to detect significant differences. A small difference in FEV_1 or FVC, which might plausibly reflect the same pathological processes as a larger difference in one of the later expiratory flow rates, could be detectable in a reliable manner with a smaller sample than would be required for a flow volume curve analysis. In other words, what is gained by virtue of the increased sensitivity of the later expiratory flow rates may be lost by virtue of their variation. In addition, prediction equations for calculating what are normal flow rates are by no means so well established as they are for spirometry.

While measurements of diffusing capacity have been increasing in popularity in the detection of interstitial lung disease, their place in the assessment of obstructive lung disease, at least in the epidemiological field setting, is far from established. Readers interested in pursuing this test further are referred to pp. 62–72 of the ATS review for an in-depth discussion on these procedures and their usefulness.

As already indicated, there are many pulmonary function tests, such as measurements of total lung capacity (TLC), functional residual capacity (FRC) and residual capacity, that might be useful in epidemiological studies in particular contexts, whether in the community or in certain occupational settings. However, most are limited to use in a laboratory or have not yet been found to contribute significantly to our further understanding of the nature and development of lung disease. As far as TLC, FRC and residual capacity are concerned, it must be recognized that there are virtually no data on these variables in survey settings, in part because of the complexity of the instrumentation required to measure them and in part because these tests are not likely to give abnormal results in cases of minor obstructive lung disease. Neither is their place in the assessment of patients with interstitial lung disease firmly established. It is not likely that they will replace the measurement of FVC and diffusing capacity in surveys directed towards this problem.

If a decision is made to measure FRC or TLC, the recommendations of the ATS should be taken into account, as given on page 80 of their review. The body plethysmograph is considered to be the best technique in that it most closely reflects true lung volumes, does not require irradiation, is time efficient, and has a small coefficient of variation between duplicate determinations.

Interest in other tests has waxed and waned from time to time. The closing volume and closing capacity tests have suffered this fate. Both tests are susceptible to wide observer variation and a lack of clear-cut prediction equations for normality, and can give abnormal results in a variety of conditions, so that they lack specificity.

One test that has found wide acceptance recently, particularly in studies of occupational populations, is the assessment of bronchial reactivity to chemical or thermal challenge. In this test, known doses of histamine or methylcholine are applied to the bronchial tree by inhalation of an aerosol. Spirometric measurements are made before and after challenge, changes in FEV_1 of greater than 20 % being indicative of greater than expected reactiveness in the bronchial response. Information on this test is given in Annex 6.

While bronchial hyper-reactivity is a feature of asthma and is found with more than expected frequency in groups of patients with chronic airflow limitation, its natural history and prognostic significance in free living populations is not known. Whether it represents a tendency to pathological "over-reaction" to various environmental stimuli, or a heightened defence response for the protection of the lungs, is not known. The distribution of bronchial reactivity in the population appears to be continuous, but whether normal or bimodal is not known.

SPECIAL INVESTIGATIONS

Chest radiography

With the development of pulmonary function tests of considerable sophistication, and the desire to estimate prevalence rates of early, rather than advanced chronic obstructive lung disease, the place of chest radiography has decreased very substantially. Its only legitimate use is in the detailed follow-up of those whose pulmonary function studies have shown very significant lung disease. It may be useful in defining the extent of cor pulmonale by providing corroborative evidence of over-inflation consistent with emphysema, or of marked air trapping due to other forms of chronic airway obstruction.

Height and weight

Lung function varies with the size of the subject. It is usual to make adjustments for variation in height, and weight may sometimes also be included in the adjustments. The adjustments may be made by using tables to find the predicted result of the test for a given height, age and sex, from which the observed value can be expressed as a percentage of the predicted value. Adjustment can also be made from a regression equation calculated from the data collected in the survey. In either case, accurate measurements of height and weight are needed.

Height should be measured on a good-quality, stable stadiometer. Stadiometers attached to weighing machines are *not* suitable, as the subject has to stand on the unstable weighing platform. Moreover, the scale is usually too coarsely graduated and the cursor is not at right angles to the scale.

The subject should be barefoot and should stand with his heels together, pressed against the heelboard of the stadiometer. The head should be held in the Frankfort plane, so that the lower border of the orbit is at the same level as the upper margin of the external auditory meatus. This position tends to make the subject feel he is tucking his chin in. The cursor is lowered on to the head and its position is measured to the nearest 5 mm *below* the pointer, unless the pointer falls *exactly* on a graduation mark. Provided this procedure is always used, mean values of height can be corrected by adding 2.5 mm; the variance will not be affected.

Weight should be measured on a lever balance to the nearest 100 g *below* the pointer, unless the pointer falls on a graduation mark. The subject should be without shoes and preferably only in light clothing. The balance should be calibrated regularly.

CHAPTER 4

Data preparation and statistical analysis

In this chapter the methods of handling and analysing the data are outlined. This part of a study is quite as important as the fieldwork and requires the same detailed planning if it is to be done quickly and with a minimum of errors. Even the most carefully planned strategy can be upset by the unexpected, but most of the problems can be avoided with foresight.

DATA PREPARATION

As previously mentioned, the use of a computer is almost mandatory for processing data from a cohort study, and it is therefore assumed in the following discussion that one is available. The design of the data processing system when a computer is used comprises the following four stages: design of documents for recording the data, including methods for coding results; design of the structure of the computer file; design of the system through which the data on the documents will be transferred to the computer file; and design of the procedure for checking the data on the file.

For many studies of respiratory disease, the main document used for collecting data will be one of the standard questionnaires. These have already been designed so that the data can be coded and transferred to a computer-readable form. Other forms will be required to record lung function and the results of special tests. Whenever possible the results should be recorded directly on to the forms; copying results from a variety of other non-standard documents increases the chance of error. All forms must have space for a respondent's survey number so that information from the questionnaire and the physical tests can be linked for each individual.

When the general design of the forms is complete, the way the data are to appear on the computer file must be worked out. The file may be made in a number of ways, depending on the computing facility, but the use of 80-column punch cards as the basic unit in the file will be considered here, since these cards are widely employed throughout the world. The coded data will be punched so that up to 80 characters will appear on a card. Two items must appear on every card, namely the individual's survey number and the sequence number of the card within the individual's set of cards (record). The record might be made up of data from the questionnaire on cards 1 and 2, and lung function measurements on card 3. The same system may be used after follow-up examination, but an additional digit is required to indicate the examination number. Additional information, such as details of consultations with a practitioner, may be added at irregular intervals. Cards with this information must also be identifiable by the same technique—a third digit might be required, coded say 0 for regular examinations and 1 for irregular consultations. The aim of these numbers is to provide sufficient information to enable the cards to be sorted into a predetermined order if they are out of order when the file is first created.

When the record structure—the order and the number of cards for each respondent—has been decided, a code key should be prepared. This is a list of the names of the variables, their position on the punch cards (indicated by column number), and their codes and coding instructions. This list should account for *all* the variables in the record from beginning to end. It will be used by the programmer to define for the computer the position in the record of variables for analysis. It is also a useful general reference document.

Data from the study will probably be collected at different times. It may be, for example, that the questionnaire is administered several weeks before the lung function tests are done. The questionnaire data can be prepared before the lung function data, and preliminary analyses may even be possible. The whole process by which the data leave the field, are prepared for the computer and are ultimately combined in a single master file, must be charted on a flow diagram. This *essential* step during the preparation of the protocol will often reveal difficulties that were not obvious before and that, if neglected, could have adverse effects on the study timetable.

Finally, when the data are entered into the computer they must be checked. Even if checking has been done by eye when the forms were being coded or at some other time, this computer check must be done. Every variable should be checked for its range. Errors should be signalled if a variable has a value beyond the range in which it should reasonably lie. These checks should include the survey numbers and card numbers. Logical checks should also be made to determine whether two or more variables have values that are consistent with each other. Logical checks can be made, for example, where two questions are linked such that the answer to the second is only given if the answer to the first is positive, or where a change in height from one examination to another must be in one direction only, as for schoolchildren.

Each stage of data processing described here should appear in detail in the study protocol. In multicentre studies the methods should be identical, with the exception of the third stage describing how the data are transferred from the field to the computer. This may differ according to local circumstances but the end results, the individual records and the master file, should have the same structure in every centre.

STATISTICAL ANALYSIS

First examination

Analysis of cohort study data will start with the summarizing of the cross-sectional data from the first interview and examinations. Analysis of such data is straightforward and should be carried out with standard computer packages so as to avoid unnecessary *ad hoc* programming.

The response rate, i.e. the number of respondents divided by the total number of people in the sample, should first be calculated. Response can be given as a single figure for the whole study, but it is often useful to show response as a function of variables that may be related to it, such as age, sex or location. To enable response rates to be calculated for subgroups, the total number of the subgroup in the sample must be known. An example of a possible method of tabulating response rates is shown in Table 5.

The rest of the analysis will be guided by the hypothesis that the study was designed to test. This can be rephrased in the form of a statistically testable model (Chapter 1), which should have been described in the protocol, should include all the variables of importance, and will indicate which relations are likely to be dominant in the analysis. In the first cross-sectional analysis the model might be: lung function = age + sex + height + weight + race + smoking habits. This might be tested immediately, as described later, or the simple relations might be tabulated first. Whether the simple or complex analyses are done first is not crucial; both must be done eventually if the data are to be fully understood.

For continuous variables, one-way frequency distributions should be obtained for all variables (Table 6). These may include all the observations or be obtained separately for subgroups defined by variables in the model. For example, in children aged 7–12 years, the overall distribution of PEFR would be affected by the number of children in each age group. If, instead, separate distributions of PEFR were found for each age group a clearer picture of the situation would be obtained. Histograms of these distributions permit visual comparisons, which may give greater insight into the data than can be obtained from a purely numerical display. They will show which distributions depart markedly from normal and may need transformation of the data to achieve normality. Tables showing mean values,

Table 5. Method of tabulating response rates

		Age (years)					
		40–44		45–49		50–54	
Sex	Test	Sample size	Percentage seen	Sample size	Percentage seen	Sample size	Percentage seen
Male	Questionnaire						
	Lung function						
Female	Questionnaire						
	Lung function						

Table 6. Example of a table to show a frequency distribution

FEV₁ (litres)	Frequency	Percentage	Cumulative percentage
0.2 –			
0.4 –			
0.6 –			
0.8 –			
1.0 –			
1.2 –			
1.4 –			
1.6 –			
1.8 –			
2.0 –			
2.2 –			
2.4 –			
2.6 –			
2.8 –			
3.0 +			
Total		100	100
Range			
Mean			
Standard deviation			
Median			

standard deviations, number of observations and other summary statistics (medians, interquartile ranges) should also be given for continuously distributed variables. The tables may present the data according to other variables, such as age, sex, number of cigarettes smoked, and so on.

A matrix of simple Pearsonian correlation coefficients among continuously distributed variables may be helpful as a guide to relations worth further investigation. It may happen that some variables are unexpectedly correlated. This may represent what is really happening, but may also occur when there is as little as one observation having extreme (improbable) values for either or both variables in the correlation. This must be investigated because, should the latter be true, the spurious association may influence the more complex analyses and lead to wrong conclusions. Correlations may be verified by plotting a scatter diagram of the paired observations. Any extreme values can be quickly seen. Whether they are removed from the data set or not will depend on a number of factors, including the extent of their divergence from the average and evidence that the divergent point(s) comes from a population different to that from which the main body of points has been derived. More robust tests of correlation may be suitable if the data contain extreme values, such as Spearman's rank correlation coefficient.

Scatter diagrams are also useful in assessing the individual observations of continuously distributed variables. These variables are usually described statistically by mean and variance, which are inadequate for a complete appreciation of how the individual observations behave. Scatter diagrams may be used to provide a visual summary of the data that may be more revealing of behaviour or etiology than the statistics alone.

Discrete variables may be presented in tables showing the number of observations obtained for each level of the variable. Multiway frequency tables should be used to calculate prevalence rates for symptoms, current illness, smoking habits, etc., according to other variables.

If one variable is discrete and another is continuous, the continuous variable may be presented in the form of histograms for each level of the discrete variable. The presentation can sometimes be simplified if a continuous variable is grouped (e.g. age can be divided into 5- or 10-year groups) and is treated as a discrete variable, but this device entails some loss of the information contained in the continuous variable.

The whole model should now be tested. When the dependent variable is continuously distributed, the model can usually be analysed by least-squares multiple regression. The results show how each independent variable is related to the dependent variable after the effects on the relation of all the other independent variables have been taken into account. In other words, in the model given above, it is possible to estimate what the relation would be between lung function and smoking habits when all the other independent variables are held constant. As the model includes height, the effect of height on PEFR will be taken into account before the relation between lung function and smoking is estimated. This method is frequently used in analyses of epidemiological data and is described in most text books of statistics (a particularly lucid description is given by Draper & Smith, *44*). Because of pitfalls for the unwary, the analysis should be set up and interpreted by epidemiologists and statisticians working together.

Although not generally appreciated, discrete (or categorical) dependent variables can also be analysed by regression methods. Maximum likelihood estimates of the regression coefficients are made (least squares estimates being a special case of maximum likelihood) after transformation of the dependent variable. Because these methods fit a model to the totality of the observations, the results are not unduly affected by cells with small numbers of observations or even by empty

54

cells, provided that there are adequate data in other cells on which to fit the model.

These analyses, linear regression, analysis of variance (including the t-test) and analysis of covariance, and even the analysis of multiway contingency tables, all come under the heading of generalized linear models. Computer package programs (e.g. GLIM) are available that can perform all these analyses (45). They should be used under the direction of statisticians because both the definition of the model and the interpretation of the output require a through understanding of the underlying theory. They provide the epidemiologist with a very powerful analytical tool for investigating relations, particularly for discrete data; until recently, these could only be treated in a limited way.

An analytical problem arises in respiratory studies in which more than one reading is taken in a lung function test. It is common to make about five measurements of PEFR or FEV_1. For the analysis, only one measurement is required; the problem is which one to choose. Stebbings (46), writing of PEFR and FEV_1 measured in non-smoking adults, concluded that for cross-sectional studies the mean and the maximum of the last three measurements were probably equally good. However, he found that in a repeat survey the maximal value was obtained earlier in the series of five blows, with a very substantial portion occurring in the first two blows. This may have been due to a learning effect. The maximum value of five for both tests was found to vary less for a given individual and less between surveys than the mean of the last three values. The use of the maximum of five removed the effect of learning imposed on the pattern of responses at the second survey.

Fletcher et al. (12) also favoured the maximum value of FEV_1, but were only able to use the last three of five in their study as the first two were treated as practice blows and not recorded. They found that its scatter about the regression line with time was less than that of the mean of the three measures, thus making it a more reliable estimator of the real trend of FEV_1 with time. The use of the maximum also avoided the effects on the mean value of bad blows undetected by the observer. They recommended that all five blows should be recorded to enable the maximum of all blows to be used. They also measured vital capacity. Using a similar analysis to that for FEV_1, they found that the mean of the two blows was more reliable than the maximum. For more precise measures of the variability of the lung function tests, the values for each blow should be corrected for observer and secular biases; these can be calculated by multiple regression. These corrected values can be used to determine which of the possible values obtained from a given test is best for the rest of the analysis.

Follow-up examinations

After each follow-up examination the response rates, based on the original sample, should be calculated. Some indication should be given of the response in terms of the number of times a respondent was seen.

Analysis may follow that already described, each set of follow-up data being treated as cross-sectional. The results can be plotted or tabulated so that group changes from one examination to the next can be seen. This method, however, does not make use of the information on change in individual levels. Analysis of individual changes can be used to define the factors present before the change that are associated with degree of change, for example cigarette smokers have a more rapid decline in FEV_1 than non-smokers.

The onset of new symptoms or illnesses between examinations should be presented as incidence rates. The way this is done will depend on the hypothesis being tested, but it will probably be along the same lines as the tabulations for cross-sectional data. Associated changes in lung function should also be tabulated.

After the first follow-up examination, differences in levels of lung function can be described and may be used as a dependent variable in regression analyses. However, difficulties arise when data from subsequent follow-up are available, because there is no obvious single variable that can describe the change. One partial solution to this problem is provided by Fletcher et al. (12), to which the reader is referred.

Analytical methods for repeated measures for cohort data are perhaps less advanced than those for cross-sectional data. Expectations of the results of cohort studies must be tempered by this limitation. The protocol of a cohort study should describe clearly what is possible analytically and what areas may require development during the course of the investigation. The text by Goldstein (47) provides non-mathematicians with a description of approaches used principally in growth studies, some of which are useful in studies of chronic airflow limitation.

CHAPTER 5

Documentation

Cohort studies of chronic diseases are likely to be lengthy. Study staff may change from one examination period to another and even the project director may leave before the end of the investigation. All studies should be well documented so that what was done or intended to be done can be found without recourse to the original researchers, but the need is all the greater in cohort studies because of the inevitable turnover in staff. The protocol is the first document. It should be written in such a way as to be intelligible to other professionals. Thereafter, the course of the study should be documented with particular reference to the whereabouts of the data and the coding methods (so that analyses can be run at a later date) and to reports and publications. In this chapter, an outline is given of what a protocol should contain, and the types of documentation to assemble during and at the end of the study.

THE PROTOCOL

Guidance as to the contents of a protocol is given below under a number of general headings. Some headings may be inappropriate for a particular investigation and should then be omitted. A chart showing the basic structure of a research project is given in Fig. 2.

Title page. This should contain an explanatory title for the project and the names of the principal and associated investigators.

Introduction. This should describe the need for the study and may contain references to other work to show the relevance of the project.

Aim of the study. This should be short and very clear; one sentence may suffice.

Statement of the problem and overall plan of study. Enlarge on the introduction, taking local aspects into consideration. Then describe in

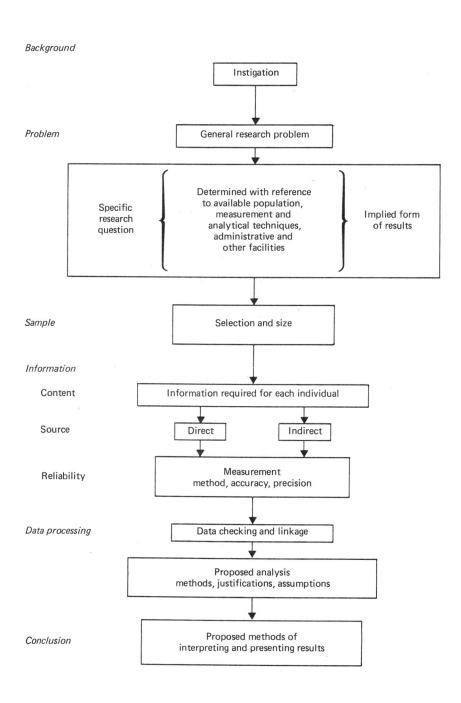

Fig. 2. Basic structure of a protocol

58

general what is planned, omitting the fine detail. This section will be read by those who do not want to read the rest; it is a summary.

Details of method. The exact procedure should be described here in detail. It should be shown that the proposal is practical and that all the likely obstacles to obtaining the data have been thought of and coped with. The population, the sample, laboratory methods, and questionnaires, as well as the organization of the field work, should be described. The use of the particular population and the sample, including the sample size, should be justified. Tables and figures may be helpful.

Survey procedures. Make a flow chart showing the different phases of the study and what is to be achieved in each.

Evaluation and interpretation. Describe in detail how you intend to analyse the data to answer your main question with particular reference to the testing of the model (Chapter 1). This section should leave no doubt that the data and the analysis will combine to give an answer. Dummy tables should be included to show the expected format of data presentation.

Application of findings. What are the practical results of your project likely to be?

Proposed schedule. Give a detailed account of the time to be spent on each phase of the study, and why. Give the estimated date of completion. Criteria for *stopping* the study, such as a lower limit for the response rate, should be given.

Facilities available. Describe briefly what facilities, e.g. for computing, are already available for the research.

Budget. Work out the expected costs for each year of the study. These should include staff, travel, durable and non-durable equipment, etc.

Appendices. Include here criteria for diagnosis, etc., questionnaires, coding methods, and data preparation methods. Give a start-to-finish account of how your data will be moved from the field to being punched, cleaned and stored.

OTHER DOCUMENTATION

Sufficient documentation on a study should be available in an easily accessible form to enable new investigators to see why and how the data were collected. The file should contain the following sections and information (where appropriate).

1. Title page and contents.
2. List of people involved and their duties.
3. List of agencies involved.
4. Minutes of meetings from the planning stage onwards.
5. Protocol. This should contain all the information outlined in the previous section. It should also include revisions of any procedure and give a detailed description of the sampling method.
6. Flow charts showing the actual progress of the study from start to finish, giving dates.
7. Details of measuring instruments (specifications and manufacturers).
8. Recording forms (including questions).
9. Instruction manuals.
10. Form letters, etc.
11. Methods of measurement not described elsewhere.
12. Coding sheets (these should include decisions made about coding unusual cases). Checking procedures.
    Flow charts of data processing.
    Description of where data are kept.
    Special computer programs relevant to future investigations.
13. Plans for analyses (completed or incomplete).
14. Publications, reports, abstracts of papers presented at meetings, etc. (Drafts of papers submitted for publication should be included temporarily.)
15. Useful tables not appearing in the publications.
    Response rates.
16. Miscellaneous information, e.g. list of schools, lists of people involved (with addresses), and maps.

REFERENCES

1. Terminology, definition and classification of chronic pulmonary emphysema and related conditions. A report of the conclusions of a Ciba Guest Symposium. *Thorax*, **14**: 286 (1959).
2. Macklem, P. T. & Permutt, S. *In: The lung in the transition between health and disease.* New York, Dekker, 1979, p. 389.
3. Sackett, D. Bias in analytical research. *Journal of chronic diseases*, **32**: 51–63 (1979).
4. Neyman, J. Statistics – servant of all sciences. *Science*, **122**: 401 (1955).
5. Berkson, J. Limitations of the application of fourfold table analysis to hospital data. *Biometrics*, **2**: 47–53 (1946).
6. Howitz, R. I. & Feinstein, A. R. Alternative analytic methods for case-control studies of estrogens and endometrial cancer. *New England journal of medicine*, **299**: 1089–1094 (1978).
7. Hills, M. *Statistics for comparative studies.* London, Chapman & Hall, 1974.
8. Roethlisberger, F. J. & Dickson, W. J. *Management and the worker.* Cambridge, MA, Harvard University Press, 1939.
9. Chinn, S. & Heller, R. F. Some further results concerning regression to the mean. *American journal of epidemiology*, **114**: 902–905 (1981).
10. Davis, C. E. The effect of regression to the mean in epidemiologic and clinical studies. *American journal of epidemiology*, **134**: 493–498 (1976).
11. Healy, M. J. R. & Goldstein, H. Regression to the mean. *Annals of human biology*, **5**: 277–280 (1978).
12. Fletcher, C. M. et al. *The natural history of chronic bronchitis and emphysema.* Oxford, Oxford University Press, 1976.
13. Colley, J. R. T. A method for measuring lung function in babies suitable for the epidemiologist. *Journal of physiology*, **177**: 40–41 (1965).
14. Colley, J. R. T. & Reid, D. D. Urban and social origins of childhood bronchitis in England and Wales. *British medical journal*, **2**: 213–217 (1970).
15. Lunn, J. E. et al. Patterns of respiratory illness in Sheffield junior schoolchildren. *British journal of preventive and social medicine*, **24**: 223–228 (1970).
16. Rudnik, J. Epidemiological study on long-term effects on health of air pollution *Problemy medycyny wieku rozwojowego*, **7a** (Suppl): 1–159 (1978).
17. *The long-term effects on health of air pollution*: report on a working group. Copenhagen, WHO Regional Office for Europe, 1978 (document ICP/CEP 304(4)).
18. Leeder, S. R. et al. Cigarette smoking in Sydney schoolchildren aged 12 to 13 years: 1971 to 1975. *Medical journal of Australia*, **1**: 325–329 (1977).
19. Brown, K. S. et al. The 1978 survey of the smoking habits of Canadian schoolchildren *Canadian journal of public health* (in press).
20. Leeder, S. R. & Pengelly, L. D. Epidemiological bases for ambient air quality criteria. *Australian and New Zealand journal of medicine*, **7**: 78–87 (1977).
21. Bewley, B. R. et al. Smoking by primary schoolchildren. Prevalence and associated respiratory symptoms. *British journal of preventive and social medicine*, **27**: 150–153 (1973).
22. Melia, R. J. W. et al. Childhood respiratory illness and the home environment. I. Relations between nitrogen dioxide, temperature and relative humidity. *International journal of epidemiology*, **11**: 155–163 (1982).

23. Kaufman, F. et al. Twelve years spirometric changes among Paris area workers. *International journal of epidemiology*, **8**: 201–212 (1979).

24. van der Lende, R. et al. Long term exposure to air pollution and decline in VC and FEV_1. *Chest*, **80** (Suppl. 1): 23–26 (1981).

25. Lawther, P. J. et al. Air pollution and exacerbations of bronchitis. *Thorax*, **25**: 525–539 (1970).

26. Orehek, J. et al. Effect of short-term, low-level nitrogen dioxide exposure on bronchial sensitivity of asthmatic patients. *Journal of clinical investigation*, **57**: 301–307 (1976).

27. Fleiss, J. L. *Statistical methods for rates and proportions*, 2nd ed. New York, John Wiley, 1981.

28. Casagrande, J. T. et al. An improved approximate formula for calculating sample sizes for comparing two binomial distributions. *Biometrics*, **34**: 483–486 (1978).

29. Cochran, W. G. & Cox, G. M. *Experimental designs*. New York, John Wiley, 1957, p. 27.

30. Fletcher, C. M. et al. The significance of respiratory symptoms and the diagnosis of chronic bronchitis in a working population. *British medical journal*, **2**: 257–266 (1959).

31. Fairbairn, A. S. et al. Variability in answers to a questionnaire on respiratory symptoms. *British journal of preventive and social medicine*, **13**: 175–193 (1959).

32. Holland, W. W. et al. A comparison of two respiratory symptoms questionnaires. *British journal of preventive and social medicine*, **20**: 76–96 (1966).

33. van der Lende, R. et al. Investigation into observer variation of the prevalence of respiratory symptoms at Schiermonnikoog. *International journal of epidemiology*, **1**: 47–50 (1972).

34. Samet, J. M. et al. Questionnaire reliability and validity in asbestos exposed workers. *Bulletin européen de physiopathologie respiratoire*, **14**: 177–188 (1978).

35. Fletcher, C. M. & Tinker, M. Chronic bronchitis: a further study of simple diagnostic methods in a working population. *British medical journal*, **1**: 1491–1498 (1961).

36. McNab, G. R. et al. Response to a questionnaire on chronic bronchitis symptoms in East Anglia. *British journal of preventive and social medicine*, **20**: 181–188 (1966).

37. Helsing, K. J. et al. Comparison of three standardized questionnaires on respiratory symptoms. *American review of respiratory disease*, **120**: 1221–1231 (1979).

38. Comstock, G. W. et al. Standardized respiratory questionnaires: comparison of the old with the new. *American review of respiratory disease*, **119**: 45–53 (1979).

39. Samet, J. M. A historical and epidemiological perspective on respiratory symptoms questionnaires. *American journal of epidemiology*, **108**: 435–446 (1978).

40. *The long-term effects on health of air pollution*: report on a working group. Copenhagen, WHO Regional Office for Europe, 1973 (document EURO 3114A).

41. Ferris, B. G. Epidemiology standardization project. *American review of respiratory disease*, **118**: 1–120 (1978).

42. Bennett, A. E. & Ritchie, K. *Questionnaires in medicine*. London, Oxford University Press, 1975.

43. Leuallen, E. C. & Fowler, W. S. Maximal midexpiratory flow. *American review of tuberculosis*, **72**: 783–800 (1955).
44. Draper, N. & Smith, H. *Applied regression analysis.* New York, John Wiley, 1966.
45. Baker, R. J. & Nelder, J. A. *The GLIM system. Release 3. Generalised linear interactive modelling.* Numerical Algorithms group, 7 Banbury Road, Oxford, 1978.
46. Stebbings, J. H. Chronic respiratory disease among non-smokers in Hagerstown, Maryland. II. Problems in the estimation of pulmonary function values in epidemiological surveys. *Environmental research*, **4**: 163–192 (1971).
47. Goldstein, H. *The design and analysis of longitudinal studies.* London, Academic Press, 1979.

Annex 1

MEASURES OF RELIABILITY AND VALIDITY

The numbers of positive and negative answers obtained by two observers administering the same question to the same people are shown in Table 1. Letters are used in place of actual numerical values, and this notation is used in the following discussion.

Table 1. Frequency (*n*) of answers obtained by two observers administering the same question to the same people. The question has three mutually exclusive responses.

Observer 2	Observer 1			Total
	1	2	3	
1	n_{11}	n_{12}	n_{13}	$n_{1.}$
2	n_{21}	n_{22}	n_{23}	$n_{2.}$
3	n_{31}	n_{32}	n_{33}	$n_{3.}$
Total	$n_{.1}$	$n_{.2}$	$n_{.3}$	$n_{..}$

Consistency, which is the ability of the observers to obtain the same results, and is a measure of reliability, can be calculated from:

$$100\left[\frac{1}{n_{..}} \sum_{i=1}^{m} n_{ii}\right]$$

where *m* is the number of rows (or columns). The term in brackets is the sum of the frequencies on the main diagonal, divided by the total. If complete agreement is obtained, this ratio has a value of 100%.

However, unless each observer confines his results to a different subset of the possible outcomes, some agreement will be obtained by chance. In the case of only two possible results, as in a 2×2 table, the usual chi-square test can be used to determine whether the agreement is greater than that expected, given the total numbers for each possible result obtained by each observer ($n_{.i}, i = 1, \ldots m$ and $n_{i.} i = 1, \ldots m$). A *measure* of agreement corrected for this chance agreement is given by Cohen's kappa (κ) (*1*), calculated as follows:

Let

$$\theta_1 = \frac{1}{n_{..}} \sum_{i=1}^{m} n_{ii}$$

$$\theta_2 = \frac{1}{n_{..}^2} \sum_{i=1}^{m} n_{i.} \, n_{.i}$$

64

Then
$$\kappa = \frac{\theta_1 - \theta_2}{1 - \theta_2}$$

A value of zero for κ indicates agreement equal to that expected by chance, and a value of 1 is obtained only when $\theta_1 = 1$, when there is perfect agreement. A value of κ less than zero indicates worse agreement than that expected by chance.

When m is greater than 2, κ measures agreement when all types of disagreement are equally undesirable, but the usual chi-square test is no longer equivalent to a test of the null hypothesis, $\kappa = 0$. This is because the chi-square statistic is affected by the pattern of values off the main diagonal, hence κ may be zero when the chi-square statistic is large. Under the null hypothesis, $\kappa = 0$, the approximate large sample standard error of κ is (2):

$$\left\{ \frac{1}{n_{..}(1 - \theta_2)^2} \left[\theta_2 + \theta_2{}^2 - \sum_{i=1}^{m} p_{i.} p_{.i} (p_{i.} + p_{.i}) \right] \right\}^{\frac{1}{2}}$$

where $p_i = n_{i.}/n_{..}$ and $p_{.i} = n_{.i}/n_{..}$.
The ratio of κ to this standard error can be used to test $\kappa = 0$. However, it is usually more appropriate to test $\kappa = 1$, or to obtain a confidence interval for κ, for which the following standard error formula must be used (1):

$$\left\{ \frac{1}{n_{..}(1 - \theta_2)^2} \left[\theta_1(1 - \theta_1) + \frac{2(1 - \theta_1)(2\theta_1\theta_2 - \theta_3)}{1 - \theta_2} + \frac{(1 - \theta_1)^2(\theta_4 - 4\theta_2{}^2)}{(1 - \theta_2)^2} \right] \right\}^{\frac{1}{2}}$$

where
$$\theta_3 = \frac{1}{n_{..}{}^2} \sum_{i=1}^{m} n_{ii}(n_{i.} + n_{.i})$$

$$\theta_4 = \frac{1}{n_{..}{}^3} \sum_{i=1}^{m} \sum_{j=1}^{m} n_{ij}(n_{j.} + n_{.i})^2$$

Other measures of agreement are also discussed by Bishop et al. (1). An extension to κ to take account of disagreements of a more or less serious nature, known as weighted kappa, is described by Landis & Koch (3).

Sensitivity and specificity are measures of the validity of a questionnaire. Their calculation requires as precise a knowledge as is practically possible of the true answers, and their comparison with the frequency with which the truth is obtained by the questionnaire (or by any test that attempts to measure some underlying entity). A 2×2 table in which the columns are for answers obtained by the best practical means and the rows for answers obtained by the questionnaire is shown in Table 2. Sensitivity, i.e. the proportion of the true positives correctly identified by the questionnaire, is $a/(a+c)$ and specificity, the proportion of true negatives correctly identified by the questionnaire, is $d/(b+d)$. These ratios may be converted into percentages by multiplying by 100. Ideally, both values should be 100%, but this rarely occurs. Values of sensitivity below 75% are low, whereas values less than 95% for specificity may cause concern. The degree of departure from 100% that is acceptable will depend on the effects of the departures on the results

Table 2. Example of a 2 × 2 table[a]

Test	"Truth"		
	Positive	Negative	
Positive	a TP	b FP	$a+b$
Negative	c FN	d TN	$c+d$
	$a+c$	$b+d$	

[a] The columns are for answers obtained by the best practical means and the rows for answers obtained by means of the questionnaire. TP = true positives; FP = false positives by test; TN = true negatives; FN = false negatives by test.

of a study, as a result of the contamination of true positives with false positives and the failure to detect true positives. For example, if a test is 100% sensitive but 98% specific for a disease that occurs in 0.5% of the population, it follows that, in a study of 1000 people, the 5 with disease will be found, 975 without disease will be correctly classified, but 20 without disease will be falsely positive. Without further tests to distinguish between true and false positives, the investigator will believe that he has 25 people with the disease. If it is the intention to find characteristics that distinguish diseased from non-diseased people, the chances of finding significant differences will be reduced substantially because 80% of the diseased group is in fact not diseased. Thus, when data on sensitivity and specificity are available, the acceptability of a test for a particular purpose can be assessed.

More detailed discussion of sensitivity and specificity can be found in many text books of epidemiology, such as that of Mausner & Bahn (4).

REFERENCES

1. Bishop, Y. M. M. et al. *Discrete multivariate analysis: theory and practice.* Cambridge, MA, MIT Press, 1975, p. 396.
2. Fleiss, J. L. *Statistical methods for rates and proportions*, 2nd ed. New York, John Wiley, 1981.
3. Landis, A. & Koch, G. The measurement of observer agreement for categorical data. *Biometrics*, **33**: 159–174 (1977).
4. Mausner, J. S. & Bahn, A. K. *Epidemiology – an introductory text.* Philadelphia, W. B. Saunders, 1974.

MRC QUESTIONNAIRE AND INSTRUCTIONS

Questionnaire

Surname

First name(s)

Address

Serial number ☐☐☐☐☐

Sex [M = 1 F = 2] ☐

	Day	Month	Year
Date of birth	☐☐	☐☐	☐☐

Name at birth if
different from above

Own doctor
Name   Address

Other identifying data

Civil state ☐

Occupation ☐☐

Industry ☐☐

Ethnic group ☐

Interviewer ☐☐

	Day	Month	Year
Date of interview	☐☐	☐☐	☐☐

Use the actual wording of each question. Put 1 = Yes, 2 = No, or other codes as indicated in boxes. When in doubt record as no.

Preamble

I am going to ask you some questions, mainly about your chest. I should like you to answer **Yes** or **No** whenever possible.

Cough

1 Do you **usually** cough first thing in the morning in the winter?

2 Do you **usually** cough during the day – or at night – in the winter?

If Yes to 1 or 2
3 Do you cough like this on most days for as much as three months each year?

Phlegm

4 Do you **usually** bring up any phlegm from your chest first thing in the morning in the winter?

5 Do you **usually** bring up any phlegm from your chest during the day – or at night – in the winter?

If Yes to 4 or 5
6 Do you bring up phlegm like this on most days for as much as three months each year?

Periods of cough and phlegm

7a In the past three years have you had a period of (increased) cough and phlegm lasting for three weeks or more?

If Yes
7b Have you had more than one such period?

Breathlessness

If the subject is disabled from walking by any condition other than heart or lung disease, omit question 8 and enter 1 here.

8a Are you troubled by shortness of breath when hurrying on level ground or walking up a slight hill?

If Yes
8b Do you get short of breath walking with other people of your own age on level ground?

If Yes
8c Do you have to stop for breath when walking at your own pace on level ground?

Wheezing

9a Does your chest ever sound wheezing or whistling?

If Yes
9b Do you get this on most days – or nights?

10a Have you ever had attacks of shortness of breath with wheezing?

If Yes
10b Is/was your breathing absolutely normal between attacks?

Chest illnesses

11a During the past three years have you had any chest illness which has kept you from your usual activities for as much as a week?

If Yes
11b Did you bring up more phlegm than usual in any of these illnesses?

If Yes
11c Have you had more than one illness like this in the past three years?

Past illnesses
Have you ever had:

12a An injury or operation affecting your chest

12b Heart trouble

68

12c Bronchitis ☐

12d Pneumonia ☐

12e Pleurisy ☐

12f Pulmonary tuberculosis ☐

12g Bronchial asthma ☐

12h Other chest trouble ☐

12i Hay fever ☐

Tobacco smoking   **1 = Yes, 2 = No**

13a Do you smoke? ☐
If No
13b Have you ever smoked as much as ☐
one cigarette a day (or one cigar a week
or an ounce of tobacco a month) for as
long as a year?

> If No to both parts of question
> 13, omit remaining questions on
> smoking.

14a Do (did) you inhale the smoke? ☐
If Yes
14b Would you say you inhaled the ☐
smoke slightly = **1**, moderately = **2** or
deeply = **3**?

15 How old were you when you ☐☐
started smoking regularly?

16a Do (did) you smoke manufactured ☐
cigarettes?
If Yes
16b How many do (did) you usually ☐☐
smoke per day on weekdays?

16c How many per day at weekends? ☐☐

16d Do (did) you usually smoke plain ☐
[= 1] or filter tip [= 2] cigarettes?

16e What brands do (did) you ☐☐☐
usually smoke?

17a Do (did) you smoke hand-rolled ☐
cigarettes?
If Yes
17b How much tobacco do ☐☐☐
(did) you usually smoke per week
in this way?

17c Do (did) you put filters in these ☐
cigarettes?

18a Do (did) you smoke a pipe? ☐
If Yes
18b How much pipe tobacco do ☐☐☐
(did) you usually smoke per week?

19a Do (did) you smoke small cigars? ☐
If Yes
19b How many of these do (did) you ☐☐
usually smoke per day?

20a Do (did) you smoke other cigars? ☐
If Yes
20b How many of these do (did) you ☐☐
usually smoke per week?

For present smokers

21a Have you been cutting down your ☐
smoking over the past year?

For ex-smokers   Month   Year

21b When did you last ☐☐   ☐☐
give up smoking?

Additional observations

69

Ventilatory capacity

Standing height [m] ▢ . ▢▢

Weight [kg] ▢▢▢ . ▢

Ambient temperature [°C] ▢▢

Barometric pressure [mm Hg] ▢▢▢

Time of day [24 h] ▢▢ ▢▢

Observer ▢▢

Spirometer

Instrument number ▢▢▢

Enter readings as made, for subsequent correction to BTPS

If additional readings are made, enter below number 5 and delete the ones they replace.

FEV₁ [litres]   FVC [litres]

Reading 1 ▢ . ▢▢   ▢ . ▢▢

2 ▢ . ▢▢   ▢ . ▢▢

3 ▢ . ▢▢   ▢ . ▢▢

4 ▢ . ▢▢   ▢ . ▢▢

5 ▢ . ▢▢   ▢ . ▢▢

Peak expiratory flow

Instrument number ▢▢▢▢

If additional readings are made, enter below number 5 and delete the ones they replace

PEFR [litres/min]

Reading 1 ▢▢▢

2 ▢▢▢

3 ▢▢▢

4 ▢▢▢

5 ▢▢▢

Additional tests

Copies of this questionnaire may be obtained from Publications Group, Medical Research Council, 20, Park Crescent, London W1N 4AL.

70

Instructions to interviewers

The diagnosis of chronic bronchitis and other respiratory disorders during life is at present largely based on symptoms. It is well known, however, that the symptoms to which an individual admits may be influenced to some extent by the exact phrasing of the questions and by the person who asks them. To overcome some of these difficulties, this questionnaire provides a set of standard questions for enquiring about the presence or absence of common respiratory symptoms. The aim in completing it is to elicit the facts and to avoid bias due to different techniques of questioning.

Training

Before embarking on a survey, the questionnaire and instructions should be studied and any difficulties discussed. Interviewers should apply the questionnaire to 10 or more subjects (such as hospital patients) who have at least some chest symptoms (since no difficulty arises with subjects who answer all questions with a confident 'no'). These interviews should be either witnessed by an experienced colleague or, better, tape-recorded so that any mistakes or doubtful points can be corrected and clarified at leisure afterwards. Tape-recordings of a series of interviews based on the questionnaire are available and should be listened to if possible. These tapes are designed to illustrate difficulties arising in the interpretation of answers to the standard questionnaire during field surveys. A series of interviews is also provided which a potential interviewer can use to compare his own ratings of the responses given with those of the group of British workers responsible for the production of the tapes.

General instructions

Before starting to ask questions an interviewer should instruct subjects to answer simply 'yes' or 'no' to the questions. The *actual printed wording* should be used for each question. In most cases this should lead to a simple 'yes' or 'no' answer, which should be accepted and recorded. Occasionally the subject will express doubt about the meaning of the question or the appropriate reply. When this happens further probing will be needed. Repetition of the question is usually sufficient. Some guidance for dealing with the commoner difficulties is given below. When, after a brief explanation, doubt remains about whether the answer is 'yes' or 'no', the answer should be recorded as 'no'.

Recording the replies to the questions

The questionnaire has been set out to facilitate transfer of the data to punched cards. Most of the questions are of the 'yes'/'no' type and replies to these questions may be coded directly in the boxes provided. Instructions for coding responses need to be defined by the survey planner before the survey begins. (Suggested coding: yes = 1, no = 2, not applicable = 8). Where the answer to a question is a number, eg the number of cigarettes smoked (Q. 16b), the number may be recorded directly in the boxes provided. Where the question is of a more 'open' type, eg occupation, or brand of cigarettes smoked, the reply may be recorded in full and the coding performed later. In some studies, however, a coding schedule for these factors may be drawn up before the study begins (eg civil state: 1 = single, 2 = married, 3 = widowed, 4 = divorced, 5 = other) and replies may be recorded directly in the boxes provided.

Comments on individual items

Ethnic group: This should be defined in a way that is appropriate for the study, as reporting of respiratory symptoms depends to some extent on cultural and ethnic background.

Occupation and industry: Details of occupation that need to be recorded may vary with each survey and should be determined by those planning the survey before interviewing begins.

Cough and phlegm:

Question 1 Count a cough with first smoke or on first going out of doors. Exclude clearing the throat or a single cough.

Question 4 Count phlegm with first smoke or on first going out of doors. Exclude phlegm from the nose, count phlegm swallowed.

In those parts of the world where respiratory symptoms are most common at some other time of the year, the appropriate word should be substituted for 'winter'. Where there is no seasonal variation in respiratory symptoms the word 'winter' should be omitted. When night shift workers are interviewed, the words 'on getting up' should be used instead of 'first thing in the morning' in questions 1 and 4.

With regard to coughing during the day, in question 2, an 'occasional' cough may be considered normal and the answer should then be recorded as 'no'. It is impossible to define the limits of 'occasional' accurately, but to provide a rough guide it is suggested that single coughs of a frequency of *less than six per day* are 'occasional'. On the other hand, in question 5, 'occasional' phlegm production from the chest is considered abnormal if it occurs *twice or more per day*. The interviewer may use any suitable word that accords with local usage provided that it distinguishes phlegm from the chest or throat from pure nasal discharge. Some subjects admit to bringing up phlegm without admitting to coughing. This should be accepted without changing the replies to the questions about cough. A claim that phlegm is coughed from the chest but swallowed counts as a positive reply.

In questions 1, 2, 4 and 5 the word 'usually' should be emphasized.

If one of the first two questions about cough (1–2) or one of those on phlegm (4–5) is answered clearly 'yes', questions 3 and 6 should be asked as confirmatory questions, and they should be asked at the point at which they are printed in the questionnaire (as in Example 1, questions 4 and 5).

Example 1

Q4 Interviewer: Do you **usually** bring up any phlegm from your chest first thing in the morning in the winter?
Subject: Yes.
Q5 Interviewer: Do you **usually** bring up any phlegm from your chest during the day, or at night, in the winter?
Subject: Yes, but only a little bit.
Q6 Interviewer: Do you bring up phlegm like this on most days for as much as three months each year?
Subject: No, not as often as that.
The interviewer should record these answers as follows:
Question 4: Yes, Question 5: Yes, Question 6: No.

If, however, a doubtful answer to question 1 or 2 or to question 4 or 5 is obtained (eg 'yes, sometimes') question 3 or 6 should be asked immediately as a probing question. If the answer to the probing question is 'no' the answer to the basic question should be recorded as if it had been 'no'. If a subsequent question in the same set receives a definite 'yes' the probing question should be repeated (see Example 2).

Example 2

Q1 Interviewer: Do you **usually** cough first thing in the morning in the winter?
Subject: Yes, sometimes.
Q3 Interviewer: Do you cough like this on most days for as much as three months each year?
Subject: Oh no, not most days.
Q2 Interviewer: Do you **usually** cough during the day, or at night, in the winter?
Subject: Well, from time to time.
Interviewer: Do you cough as much as six times a day?
Subject: Yes, more than that I'd say.
Q3 Interviewer: Do you cough like this on most days for as much as three months each year?
Subject: Well, not every day.
Interviewer: More often than not?
Subject: Yes, I'd say so.
The interviewer should record these answers as follows:
Question 1: No, Question 2: Yes, Question 3: Yes.

In question 7a the word 'increased' should be used only for subjects who have already admitted to some habitual cough and phlegm.

Breathlessness: In order to increase uniformity between surveys carried out at different seasons, it is suggested that the question on breathlessness should refer to the time of the year when breathlessness is at its worst. 'Hurrying' implies *walking* quickly. If the subject is disabled from walking by any condition other than heart or lung disease this should be recorded.

Wheezing: If this question is not understood, vocal demonstration of wheezing by the interviewer is often helpful. No distinction is made between those who only wheeze during the day and those who only wheeze at night. The word 'asthma' should *not* be used.

Chest illness: Asking about 'usual activities' is designed to avoid biases which are known to arise from sickness benefit considerations if subjects are asked about illnesses interfering with their work.

Smoking: Questions on smoking are essential in any study on respiratory symptoms. Specific enquiry is made about smoking habits at weekends because some people smoke more or less at these times than during the week, and if necessary allowance should be made for this when assessing the average weekly consumption. Those who smoke cigarettes must be asked about other forms of smoking. 'Small' cigars are those which are the same size as cigarettes: all cigars larger than cigarettes should be classified as 'other'. Amounts of tobacco (for pipe smoking or hand-rolled cigarettes) should be recorded in units appropriate for each study: the form is laid out for grams (1 ounce = 28 g).

An ex-smoker is defined as anyone who has smoked as much as one cigarette per day (or one large cigar per week or an ounce (= 28 g) of tobacco per month) for as long as a year and who at the time of the interview had *not smoked for 6 months* or more.

Ventilatory capacity: The exact procedure to be adopted varies with the type of instrument used, and training sessions are required before embarking on a survey. Spirometric readings may include the forced expiratory volume in one second (FEV_1) and the forced vital capacity (FVC) from each of five successive blows. The first two attempts are regarded as practice blows, and measurements are continued to obtain three technically satisfactory blows from which the means may subsequently be calculated. The temperature in the surroundings of the instrument is required to correct the values to BTPS; barometric pressure will normally only be required if measurements are made at a great altitude. Conventions for measuring and recording height and weight should be established carefully: eg height may be recorded without shoes, to the nearest cm below, and weight with light clothing to the nearest 1/10th kg below.

Peak expiratory flow rates (PEFR) are usually measured on a separate instrument, and they do not require temperature correction. Again the exact procedure will depend on the instrument selected for the survey, but two practice blows should be made, followed by three technically satisfactory ones.

ATS-DLD-78 QUESTIONNAIRE AND INSTRUCTIONS

Adult Questionnaire – Self-completion
(for those 13 years of age and older)

Thank you for your willingness to participate. You were selected by a scientific sampling procedure, and your cooperation is very important to the success of the study.

This is a questionnaire you are asked to fill out. Please answer the questions as frankly and accurately as possible. ALL INFORMATION OBTAINED IN THE STUDY WILL BE KEPT CONFIDENTIAL AND USED FOR MEDICAL RESEARCH ONLY. Your personal physician will be informed about the test results if you desire.

The questions can be answered by checking the best answer or by filling in a blank with a number or word.

Example: Do you live in the United States   1. Yes ✓

                                           2. No ____

If you desire help in answering a question, please put a check (✓) in *front* of the question number. You will be helped with these questions at the time of your appointment.

IDENTIFICATION NUMBER

                          — — — — —
                          1 2 3 4 5

Card Number $\frac{1}{6}$

NAME: _____

ADDRESS: _____

_____   — — — — —

(Zip Code) 7 8 9 10 11

TELEPHONE NUMBER: _____

INTERVIEWER: _____ —

                          12

DATE: _____ — — — — — —

                        13 14 15 16 17 18

                          MO   DAY   YR

1. Date of birth: _____ _____ _____
           Month   Day   Year

2. Place of Birth: _____

3. Sex: 1. Male _____

                                     2. Female _____

4. What is your marital status?
                                   1. Single _____

                                   2. Married _____

                                   3. Widowed _____

                                   4. Separated/Divorced _____

5. Race: 1. White _____

                                   2. Black _____

                                   3. Oriental _____

                                   4. Other _____

6. What is the highest grade completed in school? _____

   (*For example*: 12 years is completion of high school)

These questions pertain mainly to your chest. Please answer *yes* or *no* if possible. If a question does not appear to be applicable to you, check the *does not apply* space. If you are in doubt about whether your answer is *yes* or *no*, record *no*.

Card Number

COUGH

6

7A. Do you usually have a cough? (Count a cough with first smoke or on first going out-of-doors. Exclude clearing of throat.) [If *no*, skip to Question 7C.] 1. Yes ____ 2. No ____ (21)

B. Do you usually cough as much as 4 to 6 times a day, 4 or more days out of the week? 1. Yes ____ 2. No. ____ (22)

C. Do you usually cough at all on getting up, or first thing in the morning? 1. Yes ____ 2. No ____ (23)

D. Do you usually cough at all during the rest of the day or at night? 1. Yes ____ 2. No ____ (24)

IF *YES* TO ANY OF ABOVE (7A, B, C, OR D), ANSWER THE FOLLOWING:
IF *NO* TO ALL, CHECK *DOES NOT APPLY* AND SKIP TO NEXT PAGE.

E. Do you usually cough like this on most days for 3 consecutive months or more during the year? 1. Yes ____ 2. No ____ (25)

8. Does not apply ____

F. For how many years have you had this cough? _____ (26–27)

Number of years

88. Does not apply ____

78

PHLEGM

8A. Do you usually bring up phlegm from your chest?　　1. Yes＿＿　2. No＿＿　(28)
(Count phlegm with the first smoke or on first going
out-of-doors. Exclude phlegm from the nose. Count
swallowed phlegm.)
[If *no*, skip to 8C.]

B. Do you usually bring up phlegm like this as much as　1. Yes＿＿　2. No＿＿　(29)
twice a day, 4 or more days out of the week?

C. Do you usually bring up phlegm at all on getting up,　1. Yes＿＿　2. No＿＿　(30)
or first thing in the morning?

D. Do you usually bring up phlegm at all during the rest　1. Yes＿＿　2. No＿＿　(31)
of the day or at night?

IF *YES* TO ANY OF THE ABOVE (8A, B, C, OR D),
ANSWER THE FOLLOWING:
IF *NO* TO ALL, CHECK *DOES NOT APPLY* AND SKIP TO NEXT PAGE.

E. Do you bring up phlegm like this on most days for 3　1. Yes＿＿　2. No＿＿
consecutive months or more during the year?
　　　　　　　　　　　　　　　　　　　　　　　　8. Does not apply＿＿　(32)

F. For how many years have you had trouble with
phlegm?　　　　　　　　　　　　　　　　　＿＿＿＿＿＿＿＿＿＿＿
　　　　　　　　　　　　　　　　　　　　　　Number of years

　　　　　　　　　　　　　　　　　　　88. Does not apply＿＿　(33–34)

EPISODES OF COUGH AND PHLEGM

9A. Have you had periods or episodes of (increased*)   1. Yes＿＿   2. No＿＿   (35)
cough and phlegm lasting for 3 weeks or more each
year?
* (For persons who usually have cough and/or phlegm)

＿＿＿ IF *YES* TO 9A: ＿＿＿＿＿＿＿＿＿

B. For how long have you had at least 1 such episode per   ＿＿＿＿＿＿＿＿   (36–37)
year?   Number of years

     88. Does not apply ＿＿＿＿

WHEEZING

10A. Does your chest ever sound wheezy or whistling:

     1. When you have a cold?   1. Yes＿＿   2. No＿＿   (38)

     2. Occasionally apart from colds?   1. Yes＿＿   2. No＿＿   (39)

     3. Most days or nights   1. Yes＿＿   2. No＿＿   (40)

＿＿＿ IF *YES* TO 1, 2, OR 3 IN 10A: ＿＿＿＿＿＿＿

B. For how many years has this been present?   ＿＿＿＿＿＿＿＿   (41–42)
     Number of years

     88. Does not apply ＿＿＿＿

11A. Have you ever had an attack of wheezing that has made
you feel short of breath?   1. Yes＿＿   2. No＿＿   (43)

＿＿＿ IF *YES* TO 11A: ＿＿＿＿＿＿＿

B. How old were you when you had your first   ＿＿＿Age in years   (44–45)
such attack?   88. Does not apply ＿＿＿＿

C. Have you had 2 or more such episodes?   1. Yes＿＿   2. No＿＿   (46)
     8. Does not apply ＿＿＿＿

D. Have you ever required medicine or treatment   1. Yes＿＿   2. No＿＿   (47)
for the(se) attack(s)?   88. Does not apply ＿＿＿＿

80

BREATHLESSNESS

12. If disabled from walking by any condition other than heart or lung disease, please describe and proceed to Question 14A.

Nature of condition(s): ————————————————— (48)

13A. Are you troubled by shortness of breath when hurrying on the level or walking up a slight hill?   1. Yes ____   2. No ____   (49)

_____ IF *YES* TO 13A: _____

B. Do you have to walk slower than people of your age on the level because of breathlessness?   1. Yes ____   2. No ____   (50)
8. Does not apply _____

C. Do you ever have to stop for breath when walking at your own pace on the level?   1. Yes ____   2. No ____   (51)
8. Does not apply _____

D. Do you ever have to stop for breath after walking about 100 yards (or after a few minutes) on the level?   1. Yes ____   2. No ____   (52)
8. Does not apply _____

E. Are you too breathless to leave the house or breathless on dressing or undressing?   1. Yes ____   2. No ____   (53)
8. Does not apply _____

CHEST COLDS AND CHEST ILLNESSES

14A. If you get a cold, does it *usually* go to your chest? (Usually means more than ½ the time.)

1. Yes ____   2. No ____   (54)

3. Don't get colds ____

15A. During the past 3 years, have you had any chest illnesses that have kept you off work, indoors at home, or in bed?

1. Yes ____   2. No ____   (55)

___ IF *YES* TO 15A: _____

B. Did you produce phlegm with any of these chest illnesses?

1. Yes ____   2. No ____   (56)

8. Does not apply ____

C. In the last 3 years, how many such illnesses, with (increased) phlegm, did you have which lasted a week or more?

____ Number of illnesses

____ No such illnesses   (57)

8. Does not apply ____

PAST ILLNESSES

16.   Did you have any lung trouble before the age of 16?

1. Yes ____   2. No ____   (58)

17.   Have you ever had any of the following?

1A. Attacks of bronchitis?

1. Yes ____   2. No ____   (59)

___ IF *YES* TO 1A: _____

B. Was it confirmed by a doctor?

1. Yes ____   2. No ____   (60)

8. Does not apply ____

C. At what age was your first attack?

____ Age in years   (61–62)

88. Does not apply ____

2A. Pneumonia (include bronchopneumonia)?   1. Yes ____ 2. No ____   (63)

___ IF *YES* TO 2A:
  B. Was it confirmed by a doctor?   1. Yes ____ 2. No ____   (64)
                                       8. Does not apply ____

  C. At what age did you first have it?   ____ Age in years   (65-66)
                                       88. Does not apply ____

3A. Hay fever?   1. Yes ____ 2. No ____   (67)

___ IF *YES* TO 3A:
  B. Was it confirmed by a doctor?   1. Yes ____ 2. No ____   (68)
                                       8. Does not apply ____

  C. At what age did it start?   ____ Age in years   (69-70)
                                   88. Does not apply ____

18A. Have you ever had chronic bronchitis?   1. Yes ____ 2. No ____   (71)

___ IF *YES* TO 18A:
  B. Do you still have it?   1. Yes ____ 2. No ____   (72)
                               8. Does not apply ____

  C. Was it confirmed by a doctor?   1. Yes ____ 2. No ____   (73)
                                       8. Does not apply ____

  D. At what age did it start?   ____ Age in years   (74-75)
                                   88. Does not apply ____

19A. Have you ever had emphysema?   1. Yes ____ 2. No ____   (76)

___ IF *YES* TO 19A:
  B. Do you still have it?   1. Yes ____ 2. No ____   (77)
                               8. Does not apply ____

  C. Was it confirmed by a doctor?   1. Yes ____ 2. No ____   (78)
                                       8. Does not apply ____

  D. At what age did it start?   ____ Age in years   (79-80)
                                   88. Does not apply ____

Card Number

$\dfrac{3}{6}$

20A. Have you ever had asthma? 1. Yes ____ 2. No ____ (7)

IF *YES* TO 20A:

B. Do you still have it? 1. Yes ____ 2. No ____ (8)

8. Does not apply ____

C. Was it confirmed by a doctor? 1. Yes ____ 2. No ____ (9)

8. Does not apply ____

D. At what age did it start? ____ Age in years (10–11)

88. Does not apply ____

E. If you no longer have it, at what age did it stop? ____ Age stopped (12–13)

88. Does not apply ____

21. Have you ever had:

A. Any other chest illness? 1. Yes ____ 2. No ____ (14)

If *yes,* please specify _____

B. Any chest operations? 1. Yes ____ 2. No ____ (15)

If *yes,* please specify _____

C. Any chest injuries? 1. Yes ____ 2. No ____ (16)

If *yes,* please specify _____

22A. Has a doctor ever told you that you had heart trouble? 1. Yes ____ 2. No ____ (17)

IF *YES* TO 22A:

B. Have you ever had treatment for heart trouble in the past 10 years? 1. Yes ____ 2. No ____ (18)

8. Does not apply ____

23A. Has a doctor ever told you that you had high blood pressure? 1. Yes ____ 2. No ____ (19)

IF *YES* TO 23A:

B. Have you had any treatment for high blood pressure (hypertension) in the past 10 years? 1. Yes ____ 2. No ____ (20)

8. Does not apply ____

84

OCCUPATIONAL HISTORY

24A. Have you ever worked full time (30 hours per week or more) for 6 months or more?   1. Yes _____ 2. No _____   (21)

_____ IF *YES* TO 24A: _____

B. Have you ever worked for a year or more in any dusty job   1. Yes _____ 2. No _____   (22)

    8. Does not apply _____

Specify job/industry _____ Total years worked _____   (23–24)

Was dust exposure: 1. Mild _____   2. Moderate _____   3. Severe _____?   (25)

C. Have you ever been exposed to gas or chemical fumes in your work?   1. Yes _____ 2. No _____   (26)

Specify job/industry _____ Total years worked _____   (27–28)

Was exposure: 1. Mild _____   2. Moderate _____   3. Severe _____?   (29)

D. What has been your usual occupation or job – the one you have worked at the longest?

1. Job-occupation: _____   (30–31)

2. Number of years employed in this occupation: _____

3. Position-job title: _____

4. Business, field, or industry: _____

TOBACCO SMOKING

25A. Have you ever smoked cigarettes? (*No* means less than 20 packs of cigarettes or 12 oz of tobacco in a lifetime or less than 1 cigarette a day for 1 year.

1. Yes ____ 2. No ____   (32)

IF *YES* TO 25A:

B. Do you now smoke cigarettes (as of 1 month ago)?

1. Yes ____ 2. No ____   (33)

8. Does not apply ____

C. How old were you when you first started regular cigarette smoking?

____ Age in years   (34–35)

88. Does not apply ____

D. If you have stopped smoking cigarettes completely, how old were you when you stopped?

____ Age stopped   (36–37)

Check if still smoking ____

88. Does not apply ____

E. How many cigarettes do you smoke per day now?

____ Cigarettes per day   (38–39)

88. Does not apply ____

F. On the average of the entire time you smoked, how many cigarettes did you smoke per day?

____ Cigarettes per day   (40–41)

88. Does not apply ____

G. Do or did you inhale the cigarette smoke?

1. Does not apply ____   (42)

2. Not at all ____

3. Slightly ____

4. Moderately ____

5. Deeply ____

26A. Have you ever smoked a pipe regularly?　　　　　1. Yes＿＿　2. No＿＿　(43)
(*Yes* means more than 12 oz of tobacco in a lifetime.)

＿＿ IF *YES* TO 26A: ＿＿

FOR PERSONS WHO HAVE EVER SMOKED A PIPE:

B. 1. How old were you when you started to smoke a pipe　　＿＿＿　(44–45)
regularly?　　　　　　　　　　　　　　　　　　　　　Age

2. If you have stopped smoking a pipe completely,　　＿＿ Age stopped　(46–47)
how old were you when you stopped?

Check if still
smoking pipe ＿＿

88. Does not apply ＿＿

C. On the average over the entire time you smoked a pipe, how much pipe tobacco did you
smoke per week?

＿＿ oz per week (a standard
pouch of tobacco contains 1½ oz)　(48–49)

D. How much pipe tobacco are you smoking now?　　　＿＿ oz per week.

88. Not currently smoking a pipe ＿＿　(50–51)

E. Do you or did you inhale the pipe smoke?

1. Never smoked ＿＿　(52)

2. Not at all ＿＿

3. Slightly ＿＿

4. Moderately ＿＿

5. Deeply ＿＿

87

27A. Have you ever smoked cigars regularly?   1. Yes＿＿ 2. No＿＿　(53)
(*Yes* means more than 1 cigar a week for a year.)

＿＿ IF *YES* TO 27A: ＿＿＿＿＿＿＿＿＿＿＿＿＿＿＿

FOR PERSONS WHO HAVE EVER SMOKED CIGARS:

B. 1. How old were you when you started smoking cigars
regularly?   Age　(54–55)

   2. If you have stopped smoking cigars completely, how
old were you when you stopped?   ＿＿Age stopped　(56–57)

                                            Check if still
smoking cigars＿＿

                                        88. Does not apply＿＿

C. On the average, over the entire time you smoked cigars,   ＿＿cigars per week　(58–59)
how many cigars did you smoke per week?   88. Does not apply＿＿

D. How many cigars are you smoking per week now?   ＿＿Cigars per week　(60–61)
                    88. Check if not smoking cigars currently ＿＿

E. Do or did you inhale the cigar smoke?   1. Never smoked ＿＿　(62)

                                         2. Not at all ＿＿

                                         3. Slightly ＿＿

                                         4. Moderately ＿＿

                                         5. Deeply ＿＿

FAMILY HISTORY

28. Were either of your natural parents ever told by a doctor that they had a chronic lung condition such as:

	FATHER			MOTHER			
	1. YES	2. NO	3. DON'T KNOW	1. YES	2. NO	3. DON'T KNOW	
A. Chronic bronchitis?	___	___	___	___	___	___	(63) (64)
B. Emphysema?	___	___	___	___	___	___	(65) (66)
C. Asthma?	___	___	___	___	___	___	(67) (68)
D. Lung cancer?	___	___	___	___	___	___	(69) (70)
E. Other chest conditions?	___	___	___	___	___	___	(71) (72)

29A. Is parent currently alive?

___ ___ ___ | ___ ___ ___   (73) (74)

B. Please Specify

	FATHER	MOTHER	
	____ Age if living	____ Age if living	(75) (76)
	____ Age at death	____ Age at death	(77) (78)
	8. Don't know____	8. Don't know ____	

C. Please specify cause of death.

_____ | _____   (79) (80)

89

Instructions for use of the adult questionnaire

The format of this new ATS-DLD-78 Questionnaire is such that it can be used with little modification of the covering page as a self-completion form or as a personal interview form of questionnaire. The instructions, therefore, are set out in 2 parts. Part I refers to the general training of interviewers and procedures to be employed. Part II refers specifically to the questions on the questionnaire, both the methods for asking them (in terms of specific probes) and the coding of the responses as they apply to both the self-completed and interviewer-completed versions.

Part I. Interviewer training

In the past interviewers have ranged from physicians specifically trained and identified as pulmonary disease experts to lay persons with little formal training beyond high school graduation. For the most part interviewers should be articulate, able to read the questions out loud easily, and able to follow the instructions. Although the data are only suggestive, the physician expert may be the worst choice to be the interviewer. There are 2 reasons for this: (*1*) the subject's desire to please the physician, which is a well-recognized phenomenon, and (*2*) the physician's inability to keep his/her "clinical judgment" out of assessing the subject's responses. If the physician can force himself/herself to act as a lay interviewer, an excess reporting of symptoms can be minimized.

Training of the interviewers requires that they be given the questionnaire and instructions to study for several days. They must become familiar with the flow of questions. Then, they must observe trained interviewers in the process of interviewing both normal and symptomatic subjects. They must practice the interviewing among themselves, and then observe or participate in interviews in which several observers code the responses. Discrepancies in coding must be reviewed and discussed. Recordings of interviews can be useful in allowing trainees to review the same interview several times. The process of practicing and becoming accustomed to the questionnaire takes from 1 week to 10 days before interviewers can conduct independent interviews. If multiple interviewers are used in any study, subjects should be assigned randomly to each interviewer and the interviewer identification should be recorded on the questionnaire along with the time required to conduct the interview. Analyses of completed interviews should include analyses of several sets of questions between interviewers to exclude the possibility of bias in assessment.

Part II. Specific instructions on the use of the required questions

This new form is precoded and the codes appear on the questionnaire for almost all the questions. This means that shortly after completing each interview, the interviewer can complete the coding, thereby automatically checking for completeness. This coding must be checked by another person to ensure completeness and accuracy before being given to a keypuncher, where it is to be punched and must be verified.

The preamble printed on the questionnaire should be read to the subject.

Use the exact wording of each question. If the respondent expresses doubt as to the meaning of the question, repeat it exactly. Emphasizing individual words or phrases often makes the meaning clear. Further explanation may be needed, but do not cross-examine the respondent. When after brief explanation doubt remains as to whether the answer should be *yes* or *no*, the answer should be recorded as *no*.

Some questions may need additional clarification as follows:

7. COUGH (Col 21):
   If respondent answers *no* to 7A, skip 7B, but 7C and 7D must be asked of all respondents. Do not ask questions 7E and 7F, unless there is a positive response to 1 of the previous questions. For question 7F, record actual number of years. (use 9 or 99 where appropriate if answer to question is unknown.)

8. PHLEGM (Col 28):
   If respondent answers *no* to 8A, skip 8B, but ask 8C and 8D of all respondents. Emphasis should be placed upon phlegm as coming up from the chest and post-nasal discharge is discounted. This may be determined by: "Do you raise it up from your lungs, or do you merely clear it from your throat?" Some subjects admit to bringing up phlegm without admitting to cough. This claim

should be accepted without changing the replies to "cough." Phlegm coughed up from the chest but swallowed counts as positive. Include, if volunteered, phlegm with first smoke or "on first going out-doors." Do not ask questions 8E and 8F unless there is a positive response to 1 of the previous questions. For question 8F, record actual number of years.

DEFINITIONS:

3 months ("E" under cough and phlegm) means 3 consecutive months. "On getting up" ("C" under cough and phlegm) may be at night for night workers.

9. EPISODES OF COUGH AND PHLEGM (Col 35):

This question is to identify persons with exacerbations of their symptoms. They may or may not have lost time from work or been confined to their homes (see question 15). For question 9B, record actual number of years.

10. WHEEZING (Col 38):

This question is intended to identify subjects who have occasional and/or frequent wheezing. Those questions pertaining to asthma are asked in questions 11 and 20, but these questions may check that diagnosis. Subjects may confuse wheezing with snoring or bubbling sounds in the chest; a demonstration "wheeze" will help if further clarification is requested. Can ask, "Does your husband (or wife) regularly complain of your wheezing (not snoring) at night?" Ask 2 parts of question A of everyone; do not ask 10A3 or 10B if answers to 10A1 and 10A2 are *no.*

12, 13. BREATHLESSNESS (Col 48–49):

If a subject volunteers that he is disabled from walking by any condition other than heart or lung disease, or obviously is confined to a wheelchair or uses crutches continuously, then the code "8" in column 48 is to be used and the sequence of questions (13 A–E) is not to be asked. If asked, the questions refer to the average condition during the preceding winters. No attempt is to be made to separate out cardiac breathlessness. If question 13A is *no,* skip remaining questions B–E. Ask through E if any A–D are positive.

14. CHEST COLDS (Col 54):

This refers only to colds in the head being followed by or occurring simultaneously with (increased) cough and sputum. Disregard "occasionally" and regard *"usually" as more than half of the colds.* This question may be modified on inquiry by the respondent: *"That is, do colds usually settle in your chest* before they leave you?" Force the respondent to decide whether more than half go to his chest. If he is in doubt, the answer should be coded *no.*

15. CHEST ILLNESSES (Col 55):

A chest illness is defined as one with cough or phlegm (or increased cough or phlegm in the case of those respondents who regularly have cough or phlegm). Do not ask B or C if answer to A is *no.* The 3-year time period (in question C) refers to any illness within 3 years prior to the day of interview. Record 7 for 7 or more illnesses, 8 for not applicable, and 9 for answer unknown.

PAST ILLNESSES (Col 58–80):

16 Question is self-explanatory.

17.1A Bronchitis (Col 59): This diagnosis may be confused with pneumonia or bronchial asthma. The prominent feature is rapid onset of cough and phlegm that completely changes in character for those who have cough and phlegm always and then returns to its former state or comes and goes over a relatively short period of time. Do not ask B and C if 1A is *no,* and similarly for each condition if Part A is *no,* do not go on to B and C.

20A Bronchial Asthma (*Card 3,* Col 7) is to be considered "still present" if the respondent has visited a physician for it during the *preceding* 12 months or is on medication or has had an "attack" within the past 12 months

21 Other chest illnesses or operations (Col 14–16) are inquired about to identify restrictive lung disease that might impair pulmonary function test response. Pleurisy, fibrosis, and surgery on the lung are recorded here; fractured ribs may be ignored if healed.

22 (Col 17–20) Treatment for heart disease or hypertension discontinued *more than 10 years before* the date of present interview is to be recorded *as no. Treated* hypertension with pregnancy during the past 10 years is to be recorded as *yes*.

24. OCCUPATION (Col 21–31):

The purpose of these questions is to obtain a coarse estimate of exposure to dust, chemical irritants, or other occupational exposures associated with lung diseases. If worked more than 1 job, determine total years worked at all jobs and on average if exposure was mild, moderate, or severe. For some individuals, question D may repeat answers contained in B and C. Columns 23–24 and 27–28 are for recording total years worked. Specific job is not coded in question B and C. Column 30–31 uses a simple classification that characterizes the population into broad categories and corresponds to the U.S. Census Code of Occupational Classification as follows:

Occupational Code Corresponding to the U.S. Census Code of Occupational Classification
Code no.
01. Professional, technical, and kindred workers
02. Managers and administrators, except farm
03. Sales workers
04. Clerical and kindred workers
05. Craftsmen and kindred workers
06. Operatives, except transport
07. Transport equipment operatives
08. Laborers, except farm
09. Farmers and farm managers
10. Farm laborers and farm foremen
11. Service workers, except private household
12. Private household workers
13. Not in work force

25. TOBACCO SMOKING (Col 32–62):

25A   A cigarette smoker is defined as a person who has smoked at least 20 packs of cigarettes or at least 1 cigarette per day for at least 1 year (or cigarettes rolled from 12 oz of tobacco) in a lifetime. For subject who has not smoked that many cigarettes, skip to question 26A.

25B   A current cigarette smoker is a person who was a regular cigarette smoker up to a month ago.

25D   Is asked only if the respondent answered *no* to 25B, "Do you now smoke cigarettes?"

25E   Some persons may respond that they buy cigarettes by the carton. Must know the number of packages per carton (usually 10 packages) and the number of cigarettes per package (usually 20 cigarettes per package in the United States). The interviewer can then convert the answer to this question and question 25F to cigarettes per day.
The balance of the questions are self-explanatory.

28. FAMILY HISTORY (Col 63–78):

The subject may raise some question about why family history is included. It is fair to say that some respiratory disease "runs in families" and it is important in any consideration of the kind of data being collected that a brief family history be obtained. The reason for knowing mother's and father's age and whether alive is to estimate risks of disease (for example, risk of getting emphysema). Cause of death in parents can be roughly coded in broad categories using a single digit. One code useful for this questionnaire is to consider the listed conditions as separate codes 1–5, heart disease as 6, other cancers as 7, 8 as not applicable, and 9 as unknown.

Supplementary questions

Several additional questions have been pretested and are to be considered as supplementary questions to be added to the end of each sequence of questions or at the end of the questionnaire. These are not recommended as part of the minimum questionnaire, but can be used to obtain additional details, or they may have specific usefulness in different population groups.

For the most part, the occasions for when to add these questions are obvious. For example, in regions of the United States that do not have distinctly definable winters, it may be useful to use the questions that identify the specific months in which the symptoms occur (7G, 8G, 11E, 13G). Similarly, if an investigator is interested in studying the effects of indoor pollution, it would be useful to use the census questions on home heating, cooking, and fuel sources. Finally, in parts of the country or in specific population groups in which tuberculosis is suspected to be an important factor, it would be useful to include as part of the past history the question on tuberculosis (17.5A).

**Additional questions that have been tested
and are suggested for various kinds of studies and
in particular environments**

GENERAL DEMOGRAPHIC QUESTIONS

5. Race

Category 4 can be added to in various ways particular to the area being studied. e.g.,

American Indian

Mexican-American

Italian-American

Etc.

RESIDENCE

How long have you lived in the same part of town?

_____ Number of years

How many residence changes (changes of town) have you had in the last 10 years?

_____ Number of changes

93

HOME HEATING AND FUEL

How is your home heated?

1. Steam or hot water _____
2. Warm air furnace _____
3. Floor, wall, or pipeless furnace _____
4. Built-in electric units _____
5. Other means – with flue _____
6. Other means – without flue _____
7. Not heated _____

What fuel is used most for heating your home?

1. Coal or coke _____
2. Wood _____
3. Utility gas _____
4. Bottled, tank or LP gas _____
5. Electricity _____
6. Fuel oil, kerosene, etc. _____
7. Other _____
8. No fuel _____

What fuel is used most for cooking in your home?

1. Coal or coke _____
2. Wood _____
3. Utility gas _____
4. Bottled, tank, or LP gas _____
5. Electricity _____
6. Fuel oil, kerosene _____

94

(7G.) During which months does your cough give you the most trouble? (Check months troubled) OR: Check here if no relation to time of year _____ 1

8 Does not apply_____

Jan	Feb	Mar	Apr	May	Jun	Jul	Aug	Sep	Oct	Nov	Dec
___	___	___	___	___	___	___	___	___	___	___	___

(8G.) During which months does your phlegm give you the most trouble? (Check months troubled) OR: Check here if no relation to time of year _____ 1

8 Does not apply _____

Jan	Feb	Mar	Apr	May	Jun	Jul	Aug	Sep	Oct	Nov	Dec
___	___	___	___	___	___	___	___	___	___	___	___

(11E.) During which months does your wheezing give you the most trouble? (Check months troubled) OR: Check here if no relation to time of year _____ 1

8 Does not apply _____

Jan	Feb	Mar	Apr	May	Jun	Jul	Aug	Sep	Oct	Nov	Dec
___	___	___	___	___	___	___	___	___	___	___	___

(13F.) For how long have you been this short of breath?

_____ Number of years

88. Does not apply _____

(13G.) During which months do you have the most trouble with your shortness of breath? (Check months troubled) OR: Check here if no relation to time of year _____ 1

8 Does not apply _____

Jan	Feb	Mar	Apr	May	Jun	Jul	Aug	Sep	Oct	Nov	Dec
___	___	___	___	___	___	___	___	___	___	___	___

17–4A.   Sinus trouble?   1. Yes _____   2. No _____

_____ IF *YES* TO 4A: _____

B. Was it confirmed by a doctor?   1. Yes _____   2. No _____

                                                                                 8. Does not apply _____

C. At what age did it start?   _____ Age in years

                                                                                 88. Does not apply _____

17–5A.   Pulmonary Tuberculosis?   1. Yes _____   2. No _____

_____ IF *YES* TO 5A: _____

B. Was it confirmed by a doctor?   1. Yes _____   2. No _____

                                                                                 8. Does not apply _____

C. At what age did it start?   _____ Age in years

                                                                                 88. Does not apply _____

20–A.   Have you ever had asthma?   1. Yes _____   2. No. _____

_____ IF *YES* to 20A: _____

Do you currently require medicine or treatment for asthma?   1. Yes _____   2. No _____

                                                                                 8. Does not apply _____

(24E.)   What is your most recent job?

1. Job-occupation: _____

2. Position-job title: _____

3. Business, field, or industry: _____

4. Are you still employed at this job: No _____

                                                              Yes, full time _____

5. If not working at this job, at what age did   Yes, part time _____
   you last work at it? _____

(25I.)   During all the time you have smoked cigarettes, would you say you smoked filter tips:

                                                              0. Never _____

                                                              1. Less than ½ the time _____

                                                              2. About ½ the time _____

                                                              3. More than ½ the time _____

                                                              4. Always _____

Have you ever chewed tobacco regularly?   1. Yes _____
                                                                                 2. No _____

Have you ever used snuff regularly?   1. Yes _____
                                                                                 2. No _____

Have you ever smoked nontobacco products regularly?   1. Yes _____
                                                                                 2. No _____

96

Children's Questionnaire

(for those under 13 years of age)

This is the questionnaire you have been asked to fill out for your child. Please answer the questions as frankly and accurately as possible about your child. ALL INFORMATION OBTAINED IN THE STUDY WILL BE KEPT CONFIDENTIAL. His/her personal physician will be informed about the test results if you desire.

The questions can be answered by checking the best answer or by filling in a blank with a number or word.

Example: Do you live in the United States?   1. Yes __✔__

·   2. No _____

NAME _____

ADDRESS _____

_____
(Zip Code)   (7–11)

TELEPHONE NUMBER: _____

DATE QUESTIONNAIRE COMPLETED: _____   (12–16)

PERSON COMPLETING THE QUESTIONNAIRE:

                                       1. Child's mother _____

                                       2. Child's father   _____

                                       3. Female guardian _____

                                       4. Male guardian _____   (17)

                                       5. Other female _____

                                           Specify relation _____

                                       6. Other male _____

                                           Specify relation _____

1. Sex of child? 1. Male ____ 2. Female ____

2. What is the racial-ethnic group of this child? 1. White ____

    2. Black ____

    3. Oriental ____

    4. American Indian ____

    5. Mexican-American ____

    6. Other ____ Specify ____

3. Date of birth: _____
          (Month)   (Day)   (Year)

4. In what city or town was this child's mother living when this child was born?
   Please Specify: _____

5. Please list all places where he or she lived for 6 months or longer, from birth to the present (and the number of years at current address)

    Birth year (____): _____

       _____

       _____

       _____

       _____

       _____

       _____

       _____

       _____

       _____

Current Year   _____

Number of year at current address: ____

6A. Does he/she attend day care, nursery school, or regular school?

    1. No   ____

    2. Day care only   ____

    3. Nursery school only   ____

    4. Regular school only   ____

    5. Day care and nursery school   ____

    6. Day care and regular school   ____

    7. Nursery and regular school   ____   (29)

    8. Day care, nursery and regular school   ____

B. If day care or nursery school, how many children are in his/her class or group?   (30–31)

            _____

            Number of children

            (88. Does not apply)

C. If regular school, what grade is he/she in? ____   (32–33)

        Grade (00. Kindergarten

            09. Ninth grade

            88. Does not apply)

7. What is the age of the youngest child living in this child's home?

    0. If less than 6 months   ____

    1. 6–17 months   ____

    2. 18–29 months   ____

    3. 30 months < 5 years   ____

    4. 5–9 years   ____

    5. 10 + years   ____   (34)

    6. No children younger   ____

8A. How many people share his/her bedroom?   1. Own room   ____

            2. 1 person   ____

            3. 2 persons   ____   (35)

            4. 3 or more persons   ____

_____ IF OTHER THAN OWN ROOM: _____

B. Does this person or any of those people smoke cigarettes?

    1. Yes ____   2. No ____   8. Does not apply   ____   (36)

C. Does this child have his/her own bed?   1. Yes   ____

            2. No, shared with 1   ____

            3. No, shared with 2   ____

            4. No, shared with 3 +   ____   (37)

            8. Does not apply   ____

9A. How many rooms (not counting bathrooms) are there in your house/apartment?

_____ (38–39)
Number of rooms

9B. How many people live in your home?

_____ (40–41)
Number of people

10. How is your home heated?

1. Steam or hot water ____

2. Warm air furnace ____

3. Floor, wall, or pipeless furnace ____   (42)

4. Built-in-electric units ____

5. Other means – with flue ____

6. Other means–without flue ____

7. Not heated ____

11. What fuel is used most for cooking in your home?

1. Coal or coke ____

2. Wood ____

3. Utility gas ____   (43)

4. Bottled, tank or LP gas ____

5. Electricity ____

6. Fuel oil, kerosene ____

12. Do you have any air conditioner(s), humidifier(s), or air filter(s) in your home?

0. None ____

1. Air conditioner(s) ____

2. Humidifier(s) ____   (44)

3. Air filter(s) ____

4. Air conditioner(s) + humidifier(s) ____

5. Air conditioner(s) + air filter(s) ____

6. Humidifier(s) + air filter(s) ____

7. Air conditioner(s) + humidifier(s) + filter(s) ____

13. Do you have a cat, dog, or bird living in your home?

0. No ____

1. Cat ____

2. Dog ____   (45)

3. Bird ____

4. Cat + dog ____

5. Cat + bird ____

6. Dog + bird ____

7. Cat + dog + bird ____

100

These questions pertain mainly to your child's chest. Please answer *yes* or *no* if possible. If a question does not appear to be applicable to your child, check the *does not apply* space.

COUGH

14A. Does he/she usually have a cough with colds?   1. Yes____ 2. No____   (46)

B. Does he/she usually have a cough apart from colds?   1. Yes____ 2. No____   (47)

___ IF *YES* TO 14A OR 14B: ___

C. Does he/she cough on most days (4 or more days per week) for as much as 3 months of the year?   1. Yes____ 2. No____   (48)
8. Does not apply ____

D. For how many years has he/she had this cough?   _____   (49)
Number of years
8. Does not apply ____

CONGESTION AND/OR PHLEGM

15A. Does this child usually seem congested in the chest or bring up phlegm with colds?   1. Yes____ 2. No____   (50)

B. Does this child usually seem congested in the chest or bring up phelgm apart from colds?   1. Yes____ 2. No____   (51)

___IF *YES* TO 15A OR 15B: ___

C. Does this child seem congested or bring up phlegm, sputum, or mucus from his/her chest on most days (4 or more days per week) for as much as 3 months a year?   1. Yes____ 2. No____   (52)
8. Does not apply ____

D. For how many years has he/she seemed congested or raised phlegm, sputum, or mucus from his/her chest?   _____   (53)
Number of years
8. Does not apply ____

101

16A. Does this child get attacks of (increased) cough, 1. Yes____ 2. No____   (54)
chest congestion, or phlegm lasting for 1 week or
more each year?

_____ IF *YES* TO 16A: _____

B. For how many years?   ____ Number of years   (55)

                                                     8. Does not apply ____

C. On average, how many chest colds per year
does he/she get?   ____ Average number per year (56)

                                                     8. Does not apply ____

WHEEZING

17. Does this child's chest ever sound wheezy or
whistling:

A. When (he/she) has a cold?   1. Yes____ 2. No____   (57)

B. Occasionally apart from colds?   1. Yes____ 2. No____   (58)

C. Most days or nights?   1. Yes____ 2. No____   (59)

_____ IF *YES* TO 17B OR 17C: _____

D. For how many years has wheezing or whistling in   ____ Number of years   (60)
the chest been present?   8. Does not apply ____

18A. Has this child ever had an attack of wheezing that 1. Yes____ 2. No____   (61)
has caused him/her to be short of breath?

_____ IF *YES* TO 18A: _____

B. Has he/she had 2 or more such episodes?   1. Yes____ 2. No____   (62)

C. Has he/she ever required medicine or treatment for 1. Yes____ 2. No____   (63)
the(se) attack(s)?

D. How old was this child when he/she had his/her   ____ Age in years   (64–65)
first such attack?   8. Does not apply ____

E. Is or was his/her breathing completely normal   1. Yes____ 2. No____   (66)
between attacks?   8. Does not apply ____

19. Does this child ever get attacks of wheezing after 1. Yes____ 2. No____   (67)
he/she has been playing hard or exercising?

102

CHEST ILLNESSES

20A. During the past 3 years has this child had any chest illness that has kept him/her from his/her usual activities for as much as 3 days?　　1. Yes____　2. No____　　(68)

_____ IF *YES* TO 20A: _____

B. Did he/she bring up more phlegm or seem more congested than usual with any of these illnesses?　　1. Yes____　2. No____　　(69)
　　8. Does not apply ____

C. How many illnesses like this has he/she had in the past 3 years?

　　　　1. Less than 1 illness per year　　　　____

　　　　2. 1 illness per year　　　　　　　　____　　(70)

　　　　3. 2–5 illnesses per year　　　　　　____

　　　　4. More than 5 illnesses per year　　____

　　　　8. Does not apply　　　　　　　　　____

D. How many of these illnesses have lasted for as long as 7 days?　　____ Number of illnesses　　(71)
　　8. Does not apply ____

21. Was he/she ever hospitalized for a severe chest illness or chest cold before the age of 2 years?

　　　　1. Yes, only once　　　　　　　　____

　　　　2. Yes, 2 times　　　　　　　　　____　　(72)

　　　　3. Yes, 3 or more times　　　　　　____

　　　　4. No.　　　　　　　　　　　　　____

22. Did this child have any other severe chest illness or chest cold before the age of 3 years?　　1. Yes____　2. No____　　(73)

103

OTHER ILLNESSES

23. Has this child had any of the following illnesses, and if *yes*, at what age?

First Diagnosed

A. Measles (not German)   Yes ____ No ____ At age ____   (74–75)

B. Sinus trouble   Yes ____ No ____ At age ____   (76–77)

C. Bronchiolitis   Yes ____ No ____ At age ____   (78–79)
                                                                ID Dup 1–5 $\frac{2}{6}$

D. Bronchitis   Yes ____ No ____ At age ____   (7–8)

E. Asthmatic bronchitis   Yes ____ No ____ At age ____   (9–10)

F. Pneumonia   Yes ____ No ____ At age ____   (11–12)

G. Whooping cough   Yes ____ No ____ At age ____   (13–14)

H. Croup   Yes ____ No ____ At age ____   (15–16)

I. Cystic fibrosis   Yes ____ No ____ At age ____   (17–18)

24. Did the doctor ever say that this child had   1. Yes ____ 2. No ____   (19)
     eczema before the age of 2 years?

25. Does or did this child have external ear (ear   1. Yes ____ 2. No ____   (20)
     canal) infections (swimmer's ear)?

26. Does or did this child have frequent ear infections (middle ear):

A. Between the age of 0 and 2?   1. Yes ____ 2. No ____   (21)

B. Between the ages of 2 and 5?   1. Yes ____ 2. No ____   (22)

C. Over age 5?   1. Yes ____ 2. No ____   (23)

27. Did this child ever require tubes to be   1. Yes ____ 2. No ____   (24)
     placed in his/her ears to drain them?

28. Did this child ever have an operation on   1. Yes ____ 2. No ____   (25)
     his/her tonsils or adenoids

104

29A. Has a doctor ever said that this child had asthma?   1. Yes _____   2. No _____

_____ IF *YES* TO 29A: _____

B. At what age did his/her asthma begin?   _____ Age in years

C. Does he/she still have asthma?   1. Yes _____   2. No _____

29

D. Does he/she currently take medicine or treatment   1. Yes _____   2. No _____
for asthma?

If *no* to 29C:

E. At what age did his/her asthma stop?   _____ Age in years

30. Has this child ever had an operation on his/her   1. Yes _____   2. No _____
chest?

If *yes*, specify: _____

31. Has a doctor ever said that this child ever had heart
disease?   1. Yes _____   2. No _____

If *yes*, what did the doctor say it was: _____

32. When this child was born was he/she kept in the

hospital after the mother went home?   1. Yes _____   2. No _____

If *yes*, specify reason: _____

ALLERGY

33A. Has a doctor ever said that this child had an allergic reaction to food or medicine.

1. Yes, food only _____   2. Yes, medicine only _____

3. Yes, both food and medicine _____   4. No _____

33B. Has a doctor ever said that this child had an   1. Yes _____   2. No _____
allergic reaction to pollen or dust?

33C. Has a doctor ever said that this child had an   1. Yes _____   2. No _____
allergic skin reaction to detergents or other chemi-
cals? (Do not include poison oak or poison ivy.)

33D. Did this child ever receive allergy shots?   1. Yes _____   2. No _____

39

FAMILY HISTORY

We would like to obtain some information about the parents or guardians living with this child. (In single-parent family, complete only A or B as appropriate.) Section C should be completed by all families.

A. MALE PARENT OR GUARDIAN

34. Please indicate whether the male adult is:

1. Natural father	____ (40)
2. Stepfather	____
3. Other	____

35. What is the highest grade of school he completed? ____Total years (41–42)

36. What is his present job (title)/industry? ——————————————— (43–44)

37. Does he now smoke regularly (at least 1 cigarette per day or 1 oz tobacco per month)?

1. No ____
If *yes*:

2. Cigarettes	____ (45)
3. Cigars	____
4. Pipe	____
5. Cigarettes plus pipe and/or cigars	____
6. Pipe and cigar	____
7. Don't know	____

38. Has he ever smoked regularly (at least 20 packs of cigarettes or 12 oz of tobacco in a lifetime) while living in the home with this child?

1. No ____
If *yes*:

2. Cigarettes	____ (46)
3. Cigars	____
4. Pipe	____
5. Cigarettes plus pipe and/or cigars	____
6. Pipe and cigar	____
7. Don't know	____

106

39. Has a doctor ever said he had:

   A. Bronchitis?　　　　1. Yes ____　2. No ____　3. Don't know ____　　　(47)

   B. Emphysema?　　　　1. Yes ____　2. No ____　3. Don't know ____　　　(48)

   C. Asthma?　　　　　　1. Yes ____　2. No ____　3. Don't know ____　　　(49)

   D. Hay fever?　　　　　1. Yes ____　2. No ____　3. Don't know ____　　　(50)

   E. Other respiratory conditions?

　　　　Please specify: ——————————————————————————　(51)

B. FEMALE PARENT OR GUARDIAN

40. Please indicate whether the female adult is:　1. Natural mother　　____　　(52)

　　　　　　　　　　　　　　　　　　　　　　2. Stepmother　　　　____

　　　　　　　　　　　　　　　　　　　　　　3. Other　　　　　　____

41. What is the highest grade of school completed?　　　____ Total years　(53–54)

42. What is her present job (title)/industry? ——————————————————　(55–56)

43. Does she now smoke regularly (at least 1 cigarette per day or 1 oz tobacco per month)?

　　　　　　　　　　　　1. No ____

　　　　　　　　If *yes*:　2. Cigarettes　　　　　____　　　　　　　(57)

　　　　　　　　　　　　3. Cigars　　　　　　　____

　　　　　　　　　　　　4. Pipe　　　　　　　　____

　　　　　　　　　　　　5. Cigarettes plus pipe
　　　　　　　　　　　　　　and/or cigars　　　　____

　　　　　　　　　　　　6. Pipe and cigar　　　　____

　　　　　　　　　　　　7. Don't know　　　　　____

107

44. Has she ever smoked regularly (at least 20 packs of cigarettes or 12 oz of tobacco in a lifetime) while living in the home with this child?

         1. No ____   (58)

       If *yes*:   2. Cigarettes   ____

             3. Cigars   ____

             4. Pipe   ____

             5. Cigarettes plus pipe
               and/or cigar   ____

             6. Pipe and cigar   ____

             7. Don't know   ____

45. Has a doctor ever said she had:

  A. Bronchitis?   1. Yes ____   2. No ____   3. Don't know ____   (59)

  B. Emphysema?   1. Yes ____   2. No ____   3. Don't know ____   (60)

  C. Asthma?   1. Yes ____   2. No ____   3. Don't know ____   (61)

  D. Hay fever?   1. Yes ____   2. No ____   3. Don't know ____   (62)

  E. Other respiratory conditions?

    Please specify: ———————————————————————   (63)

C. OTHER HOUSEHOLD MEMBERS

46. Are there other members of the household who cur-   1. Yes ____   2. No ____   (64)
rently smoke regularly (not counting persons men-
tioned above)?

                  If *yes*, specify number ____   (65)

108

Instructions for administering the children's questionnaire

The questionnaire is designed for both self-completion by a responsible adult or by personal interview of that responsible adult by a trained interviewer. The following instructions are for interviewers. In general, the questions are to be read as written. The interviewer will be required to substitute the appropriate name of the child, or the appropriate he or she or him or her throughout the interview. If a particular question is not understood, it should be repeated as written. If further probing is required, it should be·noted. In general, the answer to questions requiring significant probing and explanation should be recorded as *no* or *don't know*.

Specific instructions for each possibly troublesome item are given below.

PREAMBLE:

I am going to ask you some questions about [child's name], the home he/she lives in and briefly about other members of [child's name] family. Please try to answer the questions as frankly and accurately as is possible. All information will be kept confidential. [Child's name] personal physician will be informed about the results if you desire.

Please start by giving me [child's name] full name.

PAGE 1:[a]

Read Preamble to subject. Remind subject that the questions relate to the specific child mentioned.

Record interviewer's number (name) after telephone number.

PAGE 2:

1. Sex of child: ask if name is not obviously boy or girl.

2. Racial-ethnic group; ask only if not obvious or known.

5. Ask: "Starting with where [child's name] was born, can you tell me where he/she has lived for 6 months or longer?" Record from birth onward, by year, each place by city and state. Finally ask: "How long at your current address?" and record in years.

PAGE 3:

6B. Ask only if positive to day care or nursery school: "How many children are in his/her class?"

6C. Ask only if positive to regular school: "What grade is he/she in?"

PAGE 4:

11. Many people have difficulty separating the kind of fuel (gas, oil, electric) for how their home is heated. We are interested in the heating technique. Radiators generally mean steam or hot water. If someone responds with words other than those listed, read the entire list to them slowly.

12. Only one answer is possible.

13. Same.

PAGE: 5

Read Preamble as written.

14C. "4 or more days per week" should be read as part of the sentence.

14D. For 7 or more years, record 7; if not applicable, record 8; if unknown, record 9.

15C. "4 or more days per week" should be read as part of the sentence.

15D. For 7 or more years, record 7; if not applicable, record 8; if unknown, record 9.

PAGE 6:

16A. The word "increased" is added only if previous questions were positive for cough or phlegm.

---

[a] Page numbers refer to those of the questionnaire itself.

16B. For 7 or more years, record 7; if not applicable, record 8; if unknown, record 9.

17A. The question should be read to the end of each sub part, with a pause for a *yes/no* answer at A, B, or C.

17D. For 7 or more years, record 7; if not applicable, record 8; if unknown, record 9.

PAGE 7:

20D. For 7 or more illnesses, record 7; if not applicable, record 8; if unknown record 9.

22 This question applies to illnesses other than those mentioned in question 21.

PAGE 8:

23. If subject does not recognize the illness or asks "what's that?", record as *no*. Read through the entire list. For any positive response, ask: "At what age did [child's name] first have" the particular illness. For:

        A. Measles

        G. Whooping cough

        I. Cystic fibrosis

there should be only 1 age at which illness occurred. For other illnesses, they could have occurred on multiple occasions. Record earliest age.

24. Eczema generally occurs before age 2. Most parents who have a child with this condition are familiar with the word. If subject asks "what's that?", give simple explanation as above, and record as *no*.

PAGE 9:

30. If *yes*, record actual words used by respondent.

31. If *yes*, record actual words used by respondent.

32. Use respondent's words.

33A, 33B, 33C, are asking respectively about:

        A. Substances taken by mouth

        B. Substances inhaled

        C. Substances that contact skin.

33D. Respondents who have had a child who has had allergy shots know what they are. If subject says "what's that?", or otherwise does not seem to know what allergy shots are, record as *no*.

PAGE 10:

Read first section of Preamble as written. Generally, the interview is conducted with a female. For those cases in which a male is interviewed, the instruction below should be as written for the female (question 40).

34. Read as a 2-part question.

34A. Is there a male adult living in the house with this child? If *no*, record *none* at the top of Section A. If *yes*: Is this male adult the child's natural father, stepfather, or does he have some other relationship to this child? Natural father means biologic father.

Complete the remainder of the section only for those with a male adult in the household.

PAGE 11:

39E.• Use respondent's words.

FAMILY HISTORY, SECTION B

Generally, the interview is conducted with a female. For those cases in which a male is interviewed, the instructions for this section should be written as for the male (question 34).

110

40. This question should be phrased as follows:

"Are you [child's name] natural mother, stepmother, or do you have some other relationship to [child's name]?"

Natural mother means mother to whom the child was born.

45E. Use respondent's words.

For both Sections A and B, the respondents may raise questions as to why years of schooling and occupational information is being requested. The interviewer can tell the respondent that the purpose of these questions is to determine how similar or different the various families are in terms of backgrounds. If any respondent refuses to answer, do not press the issue, but merely go on to the next question.

Annex 4

WHO CHILDREN'S QUESTIONNAIRE AND NOTES

Recording form 1

Part I: To be completed by the study personnel

5

Form   1   Country ....

6   **7**

☐ ☐

9   **10**

8

Area: .... ☐   School:..

Name and surname
of the child: ....

11   **12**   **13**

☐ ☐ ☐

Address of the child: ....

15   **16**

14   Sex (tick): Male   1   Female   2   Age at last   ☐ ☐
                                               birthday

Part II: To be completed by both parents or by guardian[a]

Please answer all the questions:

17   Does the child *usually* cough in the morning in autumn-winter
     season?   Yes   1   No   2

18   Does the child *usually* cough during the day or at night in
     autumn-winter season?   Yes   1   No   2

---

[a] Questions 26, 27, 28, 29, 34, 35 and 36 are optional and thus do not have to be included in this questionnaire.

112

19 *If "yes" to either or both of the above questions:*

Did the child cough on most days for at least 3 months consecutively in *each of the last two autumn-winter seasons?*   Yes [1]   No [2]

20 Has the child *ever* been troubled by shortness of breath when hurrying on level ground, or walking up a slight hill?   Yes [1]   No [2]

If yes:

21 Has the child been troubled by shortness of breath when hurrying on level ground or walking up a slight hill *in the last 12 months?*   Yes [1]   No [2]

22 Does the child's chest *ever* sound wheezy or whistling?   Yes [1]   No [2]

If yes:

23 Has the child's chest sounded wheezy or whistling *in the last 12 months?*   Yes [1]   No [2]

24 Has the child *ever* had attacks of shortness of breath with wheezing?   Yes [1]   No [2]

If yes:

25 Has the child had attacks of shortness of breath with wheezing *in the last 12 months?*   Yes [1]   No [2]

26 Does the child *ever* have a blocked or runny nose?   Yes [1]   No [2]

If yes:

27 Did the child have a blocked or runny nose on most days *in the last 12 months?*   Yes [1]   No [2]

28 Has the child *ever* had an infection of the nose which the *doctor* called sinusitis?   Yes [1]   No [2]

If yes:

29 Has the child had an infection of the nose which the doctor called sinusitis *in the last 12 months?*   Yes [1]   No [2]

30 Has the child *ever* had asthma, diagnosed by a *doctor?*   Yes [1]   No [2]

If yes:

	None	One	Two	Three or more
31 How many attacks did the child have *in the last 12 months?*	[1]	[2]	[3]	[4]

32 Has the child *ever* had bronchitis or pneumonia diagnosed by a *doctor?*   Yes [1]   No [2]

If yes:

                                           One   Two   Three or more

33 How many times?   [1]   [2]   [3]

---

34 Has the child *ever* had whooping cough?   Yes [1]   No [2]

---

35 Has the child *ever* had measles?   Yes [1]   No [2]

---

36 Does anyone else in the household have asthma, bronchitis or other chest trouble?   Yes [1]   No [2]

---

37 School education of the father or male guardian (one answer only)   Primary [1]   Secondary [2]   Higher [3]

38 School education of the mother or female guardian (one answer only)   Primary [1]   Secondary [2]   Higher [3]

---

39 How many rooms are there in your household? (including kitchen but excluding bathroom)   [   ]   (if nine or more: *enter 9*)

40 How many people, including the child, usually live in your household?   [   ]   (if nine or more: *enter 9*)

---

41 Do you heat your home yourself?   Yes [1]   No [2]

If yes:

By what means? (tick all those actually used)

42 Coal [1]   **43** Gas [1]   **44** Electricity [1]

45 Wood [1]   **46** Oil [1]   **47** Other [1]

---

48 How many years has the child lived in this apartment or house?   [   ]   (if nine or more: *enter 9*)

---

49 *You* (alone or two together) have now almost completed this questionnaire. Add one answer only:

Are *you* the child's:

Father [1]   Mother [2]   Father and mother [3]

Male guardian [4]   Female guardian [5]

Male and female guardians [6]   Other [7]

Recording form 2

Part I: To be completed by the study personnel:

5

Form   2   Country: ....

6 7

8

Area: ....   School: ....

9 10

Name and surname
of the child: ....

11 12 13

Address of the child: ....

15 16

14   Sex   (tick):   Male   1   Female   2   Age at last
birthday

Date of examination: ....

	17	18	19	20			21	22	23	
Standing height					cm	Weight				kg

Peak expiratory flow rate

1st test   24 25 26   l/min   Maximum of all five tests   39 40 41   l/min

2nd test   27 28 29   l/min   Mean of last three tests   42 43 44   l/min

3rd test   30 31 32   l/min   Machine code   45

4th test   33 34 35   l/min   Observed code   46

5th test   36 37 38   l/min

47 Has the child understood the test and cooperated? (tick)   Yes 1   No. 2

Measurement on spirograph[a]

Forced vital capacity (highest of 3 recordings)   48 49 50   litres, BTPS

FEV 0.75 (highest of 3 recordings)   51 52 53   litres, BTPS

Machine code   54   Observer code   55

56 Has the child understood the test and cooperated? (tick)   Yes 1   No. 2

[a] This part is optional and thus does not have to be included in this form.

For recording Form 1

Columns	*Item and code*
1–2	Leave blank (for WHO project code)
3–4	Project code, as decided by the country
5	Form number: 1

6–7	Country code:	Poland:	01	Netherlands:	04
		Czechoslovakia:	02	Romania:	05
		Denmark:	03	Yugoslavia:	06
8	Area code:	with air pollution:	1		
		without air pollution:	2		

9–10	School code, as decided by the country: 01, 02, 03, etc.
11–13	Serial number of the child in the school, as decided by the country: 001, 002, 003, etc.
14	Sex: male: 1
	female: 2
15–16	Age at last birthday: 07, 08, 09, 10, 11

Remarks: For the rest of the questionnaire, leave blank when no answer is given.

17–30 ⎫	
32, 34 ⎬	Questions: Yes: 1 No: 2
35, 36 ⎭	
41	
31	How many attacks?

	None:	1 ⎫
	One:	2 ⎪ These codes are
	Two:	3 ⎬ mutually exclusive
	Three or more:	4 ⎭

---

[a] This code scheme should be followed by all the countries participating in the WHO study.

33	How many times?			
		One:	1	These codes are
		Two:	2	mutually exclusive
		Three or more:	3	
37, 38	School education:			
		Primary:	1	These codes are
		Secondary:	2	mutually exclusive
		Higher:	3	

39, 40, 48   How many? Punch the number given but replace by 9 any number bigger than 9

42–47	By what means?		
		Coal:	1
		Gas:	1
		Electricity:	1
		Wood:	1
		Oil:	1
		Other:	1

49	Relation to the child:			
		Father:	1	
		Mother:	2	
		Father and mother:	3	
		Male guardian:	4	These codes are
		Female guardian:	5	mutually exclusive
		Male and female guardians:	6	
		Other:	7	

For recording Form 2

Columns	Item and code
1–16	See specifications under "Recording Form 1" section
17–20	Standing height, as recorded
21–23	Weight, as recorded
24–26	PEFR 1st test, as recorded
27–29	PEFR 2nd test, as recorded
30–32	PEFR 3rd test, as recorded
33–35	PEFR 4th test, as recorded
36–38	PEFR 5th test, as recorded
39–41	PEFR maximum of all five tests, as recorded[a]
42–44	PEFR mean of last three tests, as calculated[a]
45	Machine code, as decided by the country: 1, 2, 3, etc.
46	Observer code, as decided by the country: 1, 2, 3, etc.
47	Understanding and cooperation: Yes: 1 No: 2
48–50	Forced vital capacity, as recorded
51–53	FEV 0.75, as recorded
54	Machine code, as decided by the country: 1, 2, 3, etc.
55	Observer code, as decided by the country: 1, 2, 3, etc.
56	Understanding and cooperation: Yes: 1 No: 2

---

[a] Not required for computer processing.

Notes on the recording forms and their coding scheme

1. Because of the number of variables involved, the information collected for each child will have to go on two punchcards. It was consequently found appropriate to design two separate record forms: one for the questionnaire and one for the physical examination. An empty space is provided at the top of both forms to print any identification or name of the survey (project no., etc.).

2. The first section of both forms contains the information relating to the identification of the child and it is absolutely essential that the data punched in columns 6 to 16 should be exactly the same on both cards for the same child, in order to make possible the matching of the information.

3. To reduce the risk of errors in this respect, the following procedure is proposed:

(*a*) in a given country the "country code" (e.g., 01 for Poland, 02 for Czechoslovakia, etc.) should be preprinted in boxes 6 and 7 of both Forms 1 and 2;

(*b*) for a given school, the "school code" (starting with 01 in columns 9 and 10) should be entered in advance in a convenient number of Forms 1 and 2. Similarly, the "area code" could also be entered[a] in box 8 (code 1 if the school is located in an area of high air pollution, code 2 if in an area of low air pollution);

(*c*) at registration in a given school, the child must receive a serial number (starting with 001) to be entered in boxes 11 to 13 of both forms, the sex has to be ticked in the appropriate box under item 14 on both forms, and the age at last birthday[b] must be entered in boxes 15 and 16 of both forms. Forms 1 and 2 must be kept paired (one pair per child);

(*d*) Recording Form 2 will be completed at the time of physical examination of the child. Recording Form 1 will be transmitted to the parents or guardian of the child, but before it is separated from Form 2 it should be checked that the identification field, i.e., boxes 6 to 16, contains *exactly* the same codes on both forms;

(*e*) the returned Form 2 should again be paired with the corresponding Form 1 and identification fields checked for comparability.

4. *Recording Form 1*. One-third only of the cover page of Form 1 is used and already filled in when transmitted to the parents. It is suggested that a briefing about the survey and instructions to the parents be given in the remaining part of the page. It could be indicated, among other things, that in order to answer a question the appropriate box should be ticked when such boxes are provided. It could also be made clear that a question preceded by "if yes" should be answered only if the answer to the previous question was "yes".

In three instances the answer to the question is a figure which should be entered in a box provided for that purpose. If 10 or more has been answered for either item 39, 40 or 48, the number should be replaced by 9 for punching purposes (code 9 meaning 9 or more).

It will be noted that, in the present system, "blank" (i.e., no punch) means "information not provided" and/or "answer unknown". It is our feeling that this is the simplest approach because it does not need subsequent coding and we think that it will not result in any serious loss of information. All that is required is:

(1) to check that the main question has been answered as requested (or simply not been answered) and that the questions following an "if yes" statement were answered only if the answer to the previous question was positive (or was simply not answered);

(2) to replace by 9 a number larger than 9 under items 39, 40 or 48 (blank meaning no information); and

---

[a] If preferred, the "area code" could also be entered after the survey has been completed.
[b] In principle, 08, 09 or 10; but for a few children in the same classes the age could be 07 or 11.

120

(3) to check that only one answer per question has been given where several possibilities are offered (take the more reasonable decision when correction is needed).

The questionnaire should be printed on two pages only.

5. *Recording Form 2.* The identification field, i.e., boxes 6 to 16, of this form having been filled in as already indicated, the rest of the form should be completed partly at the time of examination and partly after the examination has been done.

(*a*) At the time of examination, the following parameters are recorded:

standing height
weight
peak expiratory flow rate (five tests) in l/min
forced vital capacity in litres, BTPS (optional)
FEV 0.75 in litres, BTPS (optional)

The machine and observer codes (1, 2, etc.) should also be recorded for both types of observation. Information on cooperation of the child should be given by ticking the appropriate box under items 47 and 56.

(*b*) When the test has been completed, the maximum peak expiratory flow rate measured in all the five tests should be entered[a] again in boxes 39 to 41. Furthermore, the mean of the values measured in the last three tests should be calculated[a] and entered in boxes 42 to 44.

---

[a] This is actually required for mechanical processing i.e. using a counter-sorter, but could be ignored for computer processing.

EUROPEAN COMMUNITIES CHILDREN'S QUESTIONNAIRE AND INSTRUCTIONS

Questionnaire

Country ☐☐   Area ☐☐   School ☐☐   Child ☐☐☐☐
  1 2   3 4   5 6   7 8 9 10

Child's name: ....

          (Surname)   (First name)   (Initial)

	Day	Month	Year

Date of interview: ☐☐ ☐☐ ☐☐
              11 12 13 14 15 16

Fieldworker: ☐☐
            17 18

I am going to ask you some questions about the child's health.
Would you please try to answer with «YES» or «NO».

COUGH

1. Does he/she **usually** cough in the morning? (exclude clearing throat or single cough)

    YES 1   NO 2   ☐ 19

2. Does he/she **usually** cough during the day or night? (exclude clearing throat or single cough)

    YES 1   NO 2   ☐ 20

If the answer to either questions 1 or 2 is «YES»:

3. Does he/she cough like this on most days or nights for as much as three months in a row each year?

    YES 1   NO 2   ☐ 21

BREATHLESSNESS

4. Do you notice that he/she is short of breath when playing with other children?

    YES 1   NO 2   ☐ 22

If the answer is «YES»:

5. Do you think this is more than in other children of the same age?

    YES 1   NO 2   ☐ 23

WHEEZING

6. Does his/her chest ever sound wheezy or whistling?

    YES 1   NO 2   ☐ 24

If the answer is «YES»:

7. Does he/she get this **most** days or nights?

    YES 1   NO 2   ☐ 25

8. Has he/she suffered from asthmatic attacks in the last twelve months?

    YES 1   NO 2

26

ILLNESSES

9. Has he/she ever had eczema?

    YES 1   NO 2

27

10. Has he/she ever had hay fever?

    YES 1   NO 2

28

11. Has he/she had any cold in the last twelve months?

    YES 1   NO 2

If the answer is «**YES**»:

29

  12. Did the cold **usually** go to his/her chest?

    YES 1   NO 2

30

13. During the last twelve months has he/she had a period of cough and phlegm (spit from the chest) lasting for three weeks or more?

    YES 1   NO 2

31

14. During the last twelve months has he/she had any chest illness, for example, bronchitis or pneumonia which kept him/her at home or in bed for one week or more?

    YES 1   NO 2

32

SOCIAL ENVIRONMENT

Now I would like to ask you a few questions about your home and family.

HOUSE

15. How many **bedrooms** do you have in your house? (Include all bedrooms whether or not in use at the moment)

(write in number)

33 34

16. How many **other** rooms including the kitchen have you in your house? (Do not include bathroom)

(write in number)

35 36

17. How is the house mostly heated? (Please circle only one)

    Open fire   1
    Stove   2
    Central heating   3
    Other   4
    None   5

37

FAMILY

18. How many people live in the same household? (Including the child)

(write in number)

38 39

19. How many children under age 15 are there amongst them? (Including the child)

(write in number)

40 41

20. How many other people sleep in the same room as the child?

(write in number)

42 43

21. Does anyone smoke regularly at home?

    YES 1   NO 2

44

123

I would like to ask a few questions about the child's parents.

22. Is the father or male guardian living with the child?

Father	1
Guardian	2
Neither	3

☐ 45

If neither, go to question 26

23. Is his/her father/guardian currently employed?

YES **NO**
1 2

☐ 46

(If he is not currently employed, the following question refers to his last employment)

24. What type of work does/did he do?

....

.... **Job Code**

....

☐☐☐ 47 48 49

25. What kind of school or college did he last attend?

None	1
Primary or Lower Secondary	2
Higher Secondary	3
University	4

☐ 50

26. Is the mother or female guardian living with the child?

Mother	1
Guardian	2
Neither	3

☐ 51

If neither, go to question 30

27. Is his/her mother/guardian currently employed?

YES **NO**
1 2

☐ 52

(If she is not currently employed, the following question refers to her last employment)

28. What type of work does/did she do?

....

.... **Job Code**

....

☐☐☐ 53 54 55

29. What kind of school or college did she last attend?

None	1
Primary or Lower Secondary	2
Higher Secondary	3
University	4

☐ 56

Now I would like to finish by asking a few questions about the places where the child has lived.

30. How long has the child lived at his/her present home?

Yrs. Mths.

☐☐☐☐ 57 58 59 60

124

31. If less than 3 years: where did he/she live during the last 3 years, and for how long, in each place?

Full address	No of years at address
....	....
....	....
....	....
....	....

32. Where did he/she live during the first months of life?

....

     (Town)   *(Country)*

61

33. Finally, can you tell me what your relationship to the child is?

Mother or female guardian	1
Father or male guardian	2
Other..	3

         (Please specify)

62

Card Number

0	2

79 80

125

The questionnaire

The questionnaire should be completed by a fieldworker during an interview with the child's mother. If the child has no mother, the female guardian should answer the questions. If the mother or female guardian cannot be contacted then the father or male guardian should be interviewed.

If the mother is available but she has difficulty with the local language, you should arrange for another member of the family who is more familiar with the local language to assist in the interview.

Before the interview, introduce yourself to the respondent. You should remind her of the study, that she has already had a letter explaining its purpose and that it is an international investigation to determine the respiratory health of children living under different conditions in the countries of the Common Market. You should not mention that interest centres on air pollution as this may bias the answers, particularly in heavily polluted areas.

At the beginning of the interview hand a copy of the questionnaire to the respondent so that she may read each question as you say it aloud.

Each question should be read aloud without altering the wording. If the question is not understood you may use the explanations given under "Instructions for individual questions". If no instruction is given, repeat the question in its original form and do not probe for an answer. THIS IS VERY IMPORTANT, as answers you obtain with your own probing questions may not be comparable to those obtained by other fieldworkers. Nevertheless, you should listen to additional comments as this will improve your rapport with the respondent.

Coding instructions

a) Each child is identified by a number made up of four items.

    1) The country code.

01 Germany	02 France
03 Italy	04 Netherlands
05 Belgium	06 Luxembourg
07 Great Britain	08 Ireland
09 Denmark	

    2) Area code

This code is unique to each country. Each study area, defined by homogeneous air pollution, must be given a number. Within a country every area must have its own number to distinguish it from the other areas in the same country.

    3) School code

This code is unique to each area. Each school within an area should be given its own number.

    4) Child's code

This code is unique to each school. Each child within a school should be given its own number.

b) Every fieldworker *in each country* should have her own identification number.

c) The Codes for questions 1–14, 17, 21–23, 25–27, 29 and 33 are pre-coded. Circle both the appropriate answer and code for each question.

When you have completed the questionnaire you should write the codes which you circled into the spaces provided down the right hand margin of each page. *When you have completed this, go through the questionnaire again and check that you have copied the codes correctly.* This second step is most important since errors made at this stage may be carried right through the final analyses with disastrous results.

If a number is to be transferred to the coding boxes (as in questions 15, 16, 18–20, 24, 39 and 31) put the units digit in the furthest right hand box, the tens digit in the box to the left of this and the 100's digit to the left of tens. For example:-

2 would be coded | 2 |

13 would be coded | 1 | 3 |

104 would be coded | 1 | 0 | 4 |

Instructions for individual questions

1.   Use the exact words as printed. "Usually" implies five or more days a week.

2.   As Q. 1.

3.   No comment.

4. + 5.   These are subjective questions. There is no definition of shortness of breath.

6.   No comment.

7.   "Most days" implies five or more days in each week.

8.   Asthmatic attacks are not defined. The answer to this question depends on the respondent's own understanding of the words. If the words are not understood at all, describe the attacks as: "attacks of breathlessness with wheezing or whistling".

9.   As Q. 8. but if the respondent does not know what eczema is, circle "NO".

10.   As Q. 8. but for hay fever.

11.   No comment.

12.   "Usually" here means quite often.

13.   No comment.

14.   No comment.

15.   A bedroom is defined as any room specifically set aside for sleeping. A sitting room which is also used for sleeping is *not* counted as bedroom.

16.   "Other rooms" refers to rooms used for daily living. Examples of rooms to be excluded are: bathrooms, toilets, workshops, stores and garages. If you are unsure whether a room should be included, always exclude it.

17.   No comment.

18.   Household is defined as any group of people, whether related or not, who live together and benefit from a common housekeeping. Living includes sleeping "under the same roof". Paying guests who share at least one meal (including breakfast) are members of the household.

19.   Children are defined as all people under 15 years of age.

20.   No comment.

21.   "Regularly" means 5 cigarettes or more a day.

22. + 26.   No comment.

23. + 27.   No comment.

24. + 28.   This question attempts to find exactly what the father/mother does and must be answered as specifically as possible. Words like – Engineer, Civil Servant, Machinist, etc., require precise qualification so that the job can be correctly coded.
The job code has 3 digits and can be obtained from the ILO code.

25. + 29.   "Lower secondary" schooling refers to secondary schooling up to the legal age for compulsory education. "Higher secondary" refers to any education after this age (including technical colleges, etc.) except at university.

30. + 31.   These two questions are used to determine whether the child has lived in the area of defined air pollution (study area). If the answer to question 30 is less than 3 years, go immediately to question 31.

127

Obtain addresses for the last 3 years at least and find from your map whether they lie in the study area. Total the number of years spent in the area and record them in boxes 57 to 60.

32. The coding for this question is:
    1. if the town of birth is the same as the town of survey;

    2. if it is not.

33. You will probably already know the answer to this question. If you do, do not ask it but circle and code the correct reply.

MEASUREMENT OF BRONCHIAL REACTIVITY

A. J. Woolcock[a]

The word asthma is used to describe a clinical condition characterized by spontaneous changes in the size of the airways. Its cause is unknown, but it is likely to result from a variety of pathological processes. It is probably not possible to determine the prevalence of asthma simply by asking individuals if they or their children have the disease, because the word means different things in different populations. In addition, some people have never sought medical treatment and some are misdiagnosed.

Between attacks, asthmatics may have no abnormality of lung function. Nevertheless, their airways are abnormal in so far as they narrow excessively in response to a number of non-allergenic provoking agents. This abnormality is called bronchial hyper-reactivity, and its severity can be assessed by measuring the response of the airways to increasing doses of an inhaled provoking agent such as histamine or methacholine. The airways of different asthmatics vary greatly in their response. Severe asthmatics, who require daily treatment, have airways which narrow in response to smaller doses of the provoking aerosol than those of mild asthmatics or asthmatics who have not had symptoms for some years. Normal people have little or no airway response to doses of histamine that produce marked narrowing of the airways in asthmatics.

Measurement of bronchial hyper-reactivity is a reliable method for distinguishing asthmatics from normal people when the lung function is close to normal. However, people with airway diseases other than asthma, such as chronic bronchitis, may also have increased bronchial reactivity. Thus in people whose resting lung function is abnormal, both the acute response to bronchodilator aerosol and the history become important in deciding if an individual has asthma or chronic airflow obstruction (CAO). Sometimes it is not possible to exclude the presence of asthma in a subject with CAO.

For epidemiological studies, asthma can be defined as "symptoms of intermittent breathlessness, chest tightness or wheezing together with objective evidence of bronchial hyper-reactivity." This definition may change as our understanding of the disease increases.

---

[a] Department of Medicine, University of Sydney, New South Wales, Australia.

Measurement of airway response

The response of the airways is measured by a lung function test—usually a forced expiration into a spirometer from which the forced expiratory volume in one second (FEV_1) is measured. The results are expressed as a percentage change from the pre-challenge values and are plotted against the administered dose of histamine or methacholine. This is called the dose response curve, and from it the dose that causes a 20% fall in FEV_1 is determined—$PD_{20}(FEV_1)$.

People who are too sick to have a provocation test are given a bronchodilator aerosol, and the same lung function tests are used to measure the airway response. In general, non-asthmatics—both normal people and those with CAO—have less than 10% improvement in FEV_1 after using a bronchodilator.

Population studies

Bronchial provocation in populations has not been widely carried out. This is because standard methods have not been available, the apparatus used in many situations is complex, the traditionally used challenge tests are time consuming, and doubts have been expressed about the safety of bronchial challenge studies. The methods outlined below are simple, safe, reproducible, cause virtually no discomfort to the subject, and take relatively little time. Histamine is used as the provoking agent because it is a natural substance which is rapidly metabolized in the body. It is quick acting, and any unexpectedly large change in airway size can be rapidly reversed with aerosol bronchodilator.

Histamine inhalation test

Equipment

Lung function. It is important to use a direct recording spirometer. Alternatively, a spirometer with an attached printout of volume against time or of volume against flow can be used. A spirometer with only a digital readout is not acceptable: the operator must be able to see the forced expiratory tracings.

Nebulization of histamine. This is simply done with a De Vilbiss No. 40 hand-held nebulizer. If facilities are available, a De Vilbiss 646 nebulizer triggered by a gas cylinder with a dosimeter (Rosenthal – French) can be used. Continuous nebulization with tidal breathing of very low concentrations of histamine, as used in laboratory studies, is too time consuming for epidemiological studies.

Histamine solution. Five grams of histamine diphosphate or histamine acid phosphate are weighed carefully, and added to 100 ml of sterile normal saline to make a 5% solution. Aliquots of this are used, diluted with more normal saline, to produce 2.5%, 0.62% and 0.31% solutions.

130

At least five De Vilbiss No. 40 nebulizers, each clearly marked, are needed. These contain normal saline and 0.31 %, 0.62 %, 2.5 % and 5 % solutions. The 5 % solution may be kept for three months and should be stored in the refrigerator when not in use. Buffering is not necessary. Solid histamine should be stored under airtight conditions in a freezer whenever possible, as it is extremely hygroscopic.

Initial lung function

The forced expiratory curves are recorded until two reproducible tracings (FEV_1 and FVC values repeatable to within 0.2 litres) are achieved and the largest values for FEV_1 and FVC are recorded. In some asthmatics repeated forced expirations cause progressively worse flow rates. If the FEV_1 falls by more than 0.2 litres with each consecutive breath (i.e. > 0.4 litre fall in FEV_1 between breath 1 and breath 3) a histamine inhalation test is not normally performed because of the instability of the baseline value. If reproducible values for FEV_1 and FVC cannot be obtained within 5 forced expirations because of poor participation by the subject, the attempt should be abandoned.

If the FEV_1/FVC is greater than 60 %, and the FVC greater than 60 % of the predicted value for the individual, a histamine inhalation test can be undertaken. If the spirometric function is less than this, a bronchodilator test should be performed.

Histamine provocation

Details of the histamine test are described below. The aim is to start with a very small dose and then to give increasing doses until the FEV_1 has fallen by at least 20 % or the highest recommended dose has been given. The timing of the doses of histamine and the accurate recording of a forced expiratory curve after each dose are essential. It is stressed that the provocation should not stop until a fall of 20 % in FEV_1 has occurred or the highest dose has been given. A reproducible dose is easily administered with a De Vilbiss No. 40 hand-held nebulizer, and the whole procedure takes less than 20 minutes per person. Special attention should be paid to the recent therapy taken by the patient. If bronchodilator aerosols have been taken in the previous 6 hours or oral bronchodilator therapy in the previous 12 hours, the challenge should be postponed to another occasion.

Two different dose schedules are outlined – one for those who have a history of asthma and/or slightly abnormal spirometric function (challenge A) and the other for those whose lung function is entirely normal and who have no history suggestive of asthma (challenge B).

Procedure

1. Decide if the subject is to have challenge A (asthmatic) or challenge B (normal).

131

2. Place approximately 1 ml of normal saline in a clearly labelled De Vilbiss nebulizer and use it as a control solution. The mouthpiece of the nebulizer is placed close to the subject's partly open mouth. Without prior expiration, the subject inspires slowly and completely from FRC to TLC, taking 1–2 seconds. At the beginning of the inspiration the operator gives the bulb of the nebulizer one firm squeeze. When the subject has inspired completely, he holds his breath for approximately 3 seconds. This should be done 3 times.

3. Spirometric function is measured 1 minute after the inhalation. Reproducible values (to within 0.2 litres for FEV_1) are required.

4. Challenge in the same way as with the normal saline, starting with one inhalation of either 0.31 % (low dose, challenge A) or 0.6 % (normal dose, challenge B) as shown in Fig. 1. Some doses require more than one inhalation and these should be given in consecutive full inspirations.

5. Spirometric function is measured exactly 1 minute after the inhalation. It is important to try to get two reproducible values, although this is not always possible. It is important to continue to do forced expirations until there is no longer a consecutive fall with each forced expiration. Stable FEV_1 values are needed before proceeding with the next dose of histamine, and it is also important to try to give each dose within 2 minutes.

6. The challenge is stopped when the FEV_1 has fallen by 20 % or more from the pre-challenge (post-saline) value, or dose 8 has been given (see Fig. 1).

Bronchodilator response

This should be performed on subjects who do not meet the criteria for histamine challenge. Isoprenaline solution should be used in most instances because it is quick acting and easily available. If it is used in a De Vilbiss No. 40 nebulizer, a 1:200 solution should be given and 3 puffs administered. Lung function is measured before and 3 minutes after the dose. This is repeated until no further improvement occurs or 4 consecutive doses have been given.

Analysis of data

Sometimes in an asthmatic, whose airways have reacted to the histamine, successive forced expirations are more variable than the post-saline curves. If two reproducible curves are obtained, these are used for determining the FEV_1. When there is considerable variability, the highest FEV_1 value is used. The percentage change from the post-saline value is plotted against the administered dose of histamine on a log dose scale as shown in Fig. 2 (closed circles for challenge A and triangles for

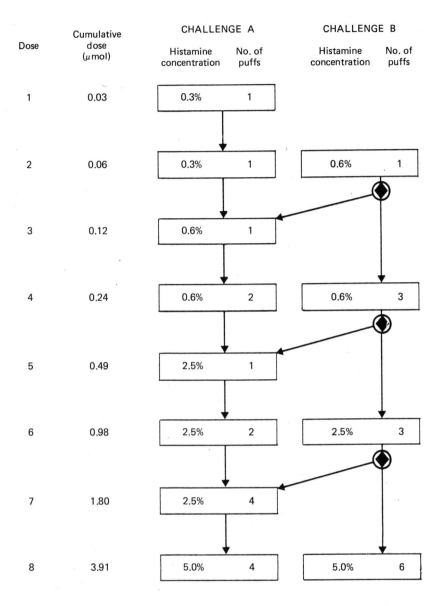

Fig. 1. Chart of histamine doses

Stop challenge when FEV$_1$ falls by more than 20%.

If change in FEV$_1$ > 10% and < 20% then go to challenge A.

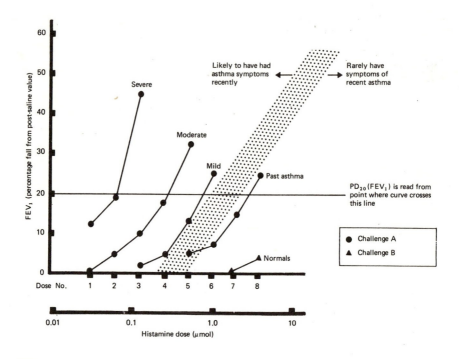

Fig. 2. Typical curves showing the response of subjects in Australia to histamine provocation.

challenge B). The dose of histamine that causes a 20% fall is read—this is the $PD_{20}(FEV_1)$. In most normal people these doses will not result in any fall in FEV_1. If there is no fall, the $PD_{20}(FEV_1)$ is expressed as greater than $4\,\mu$mol. Occasionally the FEV_1 improves after the first or second dose of histamine. Even when this happens, the post-saline value for FEV_1 should be used as the baseline value.

The $PD_{20}(FEV_1)$ which is associated with present or past symptoms of breathlessness and wheezing in different populations is not known. In Australia a $PD_{20}(FEV_1)$ of greater than $2\,\mu$mol usually means the subject does not at present have symptoms suggesting asthma, although symptoms of asthma may have existed in the past. A $PD_{20}(FEV_1)$ of less than $0.1\,\mu$mol usually indicates severe asthma.

134